Important note: While EFT (Emotional Freedom Techniques) has produced remarkable clinical results, it must still be considered to be in the experimental stage and thus practitioners and the public must take complete responsibility for their use of it. Further, Dawson Church is not a licensed health professional and offers the information in this book solely as a life coach. Readers are strongly cautioned and advised to consult with a physician, psychologist, psychiatrist or other licensed health care professional before utilizing any of the information in this book. The information is based on information from sources believed to be accurate and reliable and every reasonable effort has been made to make the information as complete and accurate as possible but such completeness and accuracy cannot be guaranteed and is not guaranteed. The author, publisher, and contributors to this book, and their successors, assigns, licensees, employees, officers, directors, attorneys, agents and other parties related to them (a) do not make any representations, warranties or guarantees that any of the information will produce any particular medical, psychological, physical or emotional result, (b) are not engaged in the rendering of medical, psychological or other advice or services, (c) do not provide diagnosis, care, treatment or rehabilitation of any individual, and (d) do not necessarily share the views and opinions expressed in the information. The information has not undergone evaluation and testing by the United States Food and Drug Administration or similar agency of any other country and is not intended to diagnose, treat, prevent, mitigate or cure any disease. Risks that might be determined by such testing are unknown. If the reader purchases any services or products as a result of the information, the reader or user acknowledges that the reader or user has done so with informed consent. The information is provided on an "as is" basis without any warranties of any kind, express or implied, whether warranties as to use, merchantability, fitness for a particular purpose or otherwise. The author, publisher, and contributors to this book, and their successors, assigns, licensees, employees, officers, directors, attorneys, agents and other parties related to them (a) expressly disclaim any liability for and shall not be liable for any loss or damage including but not limited to use of the information; (b) shall not be liable for any direct or indirect compensatory, special, incidental, or consequential damages or costs of any kind or character; (c) shall not be responsible for any acts or omissions by any party including but not limited to any party mentioned or included in the information or otherwise; (d) do not endorse or support any material or information from any party mentioned or included in the information or otherwise; (e) will not be liable for damages or costs resulting from any claim whatsoever. The within limitation of warranties may be limited by the laws of certain states and/or other jurisdictions and so some of the foregoing limitations may not apply to the reader who may have other rights that vary from state to state. If the reader or user does not agree with any of the terms of the foregoing, the reader or user should not use the information in this book or read it. A reader who continues reading this book will be deemed to have accepted the provisions of this disclaimer.

Please consult qualified health practitioners regarding your use of EFT.

EFT for Fibromyalgia and Chronic Fatigue

by Dawson Church
www.EFTuniverse.com

Energy Psychology Press
3340 Fulton Rd., #442, Fulton, CA 95439
www.EFTUniverse.com

Cataloging-in-Publication Data

Church, Dawson –

EFT for fibromyalgia / by Dawson Church — 1st ed.

p. cm.

Includes index.

ISBN 978-1-60415-044-5

1. Fibromyalgia—Popular works. I. Title. II. Title: EFT for Fibromyalgia and Chronic Fatigue.

2012

616.7

© 2013 Dawson Church, www.EFTUniverse.com

This book demonstrates an impressive personal improvement tool. It is not a substitute for training in psychology or psychotherapy. Nothing contained herein is meant to replace qualified medical advice. The author urges the reader to use these techniques under the supervision of a qualified therapist or physician. The author and publisher do not assume responsibility for how the reader chooses to apply the techniques herein.

All rights reserved. No part of this publication may be reproduced, stored in a retrieval system, or transmitted in any form or by any means, electronic, mechanical, photocopy, recording, or otherwise, without prior written permission from Energy Psychology Press, with the exception of short excerpts used with acknowledgement of publisher and author.

Cover design by Victoria Valentine
Editing by Stephanie Marohn
Typesetting by Karin Kinsey
Typeset in Cochin and Adobe Garamond
Printed in USA by Bang Printing
First Edition

10 9 8 7 6 5 4 3 2 1

Contents

Chapter 1: About Fibromyalgia, Chronic Fatigue,
  Lyme, and Autoimmune Diseases 9
  Try EFT Right Now for Your Pain 10
  Success Story: Fully Recovered from CFS,
    by Sarah L. Marshall 14
  Similarities Between Health Conditions 19
  Self-Test for Fibromyalgia 24
  The Case for EFT 24
  Success Story: Rapid Progress with Fibromyalgia,
    Depression, and Anxiety, *by Stephen Carter* 28
Chapter 2: How to Do EFT: The Basic Recipe 33
  Testing 38
  The Setup Statement 41
  Psychological Reversal 42
  Affirmation 44
  Secondary Gain 48
  How EFT Corrects for Psychological Reversal 49

The Sequence	50
The Reminder Phrase	52
If Your SUD Level Doesn't Come Down to 0	54
EFT for You and Others	55
The Importance of Targeting Specific Events	55
Tapping on Aspects	57
Finding Core Issues	60
The Generalization Effect	61
The Movie Technique and Tell the Story Technique	64
Constricted Breathing	69
The Personal Peace Procedure	70
Is It Working Yet?	73
Saying the Right Words	75
The Next Steps on Your EFT Journey	75
Chapter 3: Tapping Options and Variations	79
Alternative to the Karate Chop Point: The Sore Spot	80
The Tapping Sequence for the Full Basic Recipe	81
The 9 Gamut Procedure and Eye Movements	84
Some Optional Points	88
The Tendency to Explain Away EFT's Positive Effects	89
Practicing the Full Basic Recipe	91
Chapter 4: Tapping for Fibromyalgia as a Spiritual Energy Imbalance, *by Rue Anne Hass*	95
Three Different Perspectives on Fibromyalgia	97
Fibromyalgia as a Disharmony of Spirit	99
How to Tap for a Disharmony of Spirit	103

Contents vii

    Meridian System Imbalances 104
    The Energetic Pattern of the Spleen 105
    The Heart Is the Home of the Spirit 109
    Move Anger out, Let Your Liver Live! 111
    Tapping Is "Energy Hygiene" 116
    Healing from Fibromyalgia 117

Chapter 5: The Healing Wave 119
    The Ups and Downs of the Healing Journey 120
    Success Story: EFT on Search-and-Heal
        Missions, *by Salome Hancock* 121
    "The 'Why Bother' Syndrome," *by Maggie Adkins* 124
    My Journey out of Fibromyalgia with EFT,
        by Kristina Lukawska 133
    Persisting Through the Cycles 138

Chapter 6: Moving Forward 139
    Pain Reduction 140
    Stress and Emotional Upset 141
    Past Trauma 142
    Hopelessness and Helplessness 143
    Low Self-Esteem 144
    Secondary Gain 146
    Fears about Your Future 147
    Accepting the Unacceptable 148
    The Mother Wound 148
    The Father Wound 150
    Creating a Positive Future 151

EFT Glossary 153
Resources 159
Index 161

1

About Fibromyalgia, Chronic Fatigue, Lyme, and Autoimmune Diseases

Aside from extreme tiredness, the main symptom of both fibromyalgia and chronic fatigue is physical pain, in focused areas or numerous sites throughout the body. The pain, like the tiredness, can be debilitating. It can be a deep ache or a shooting, burning pain, all over the body or focused in one or several sites. In the case of fibromyalgia, the painful areas are called "tender points," which actually arise in soft tissue throughout the body, though the pain may feel as though it originates in the joints. Similar symptoms are often found with Lyme and other autoimmune diseases, which is why this book applies EFT to the whole group of conditions.

You may be in pain right now, as you're reading this. So before I launch into discussion of these disorders, let's go right to what really matters: reducing your pain. We are now going to try EFT together. I'd like you to have the experience of how successful EFT can be in reducing pain.

Try EFT Right Now for Your Pain

EFT is a very simple procedure. Its very simplicity has prompted skepticism from some people, but many scientific studies, including with fibromyalgia patients, have proven its effectiveness. It usually works fast and reliably. EFT involves thinking about the problems that bother you, whether they're physical problems like pain, or psychological problems characterized by anxiety or depression. It has you combine thinking about the problem with a statement of self-acceptance. This is called the "Setup Statement." An example of a simple Setup Statement might be, "Even though I have this stabbing pain in my right shoulder, I deeply and completely accept myself." While you're focused on the problem, you then lightly tap some acupressure points (called acupoints, for short) with your fingertips. The reason EFT works so well is that the acupoint stimulation soothes you and reduces the stress you feel about the problem.

Let's get started with your first EFT session! This exercise will take about twenty minutes.

First, pick a spot in your body where the pain is the worst at this very moment. Write down in the blank below the exact location of the spot you picked.

Precisely where the pain is located in my body: _____.

Next, rate how bad your pain is on a scale of 0 to 10, with 0 being no pain, and 10 being the worst pain imaginable. Circle the number below.

About Fibromyalgia and Chronic Fatigue   11

My pain before my first round of EFT:

No Pain — 0 1 2 3 4 5 6 7 8 9 10 — Maximum Pain

Now let's create a Setup Statement:

Even though I have this pain in _____
[name the exact body location you wrote down],
I deeply and completely accept myself.

Say this three times while tapping on the side of your hand. In EFT, we call this the Karate Chop point, for obvious reasons. This is the first of the points we tap in the EFT routine.

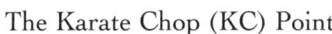

The Karate Chop (KC) Point

Now look at the accompanying illustration of the other main EFT acupoints. Tap lightly with two fingertips

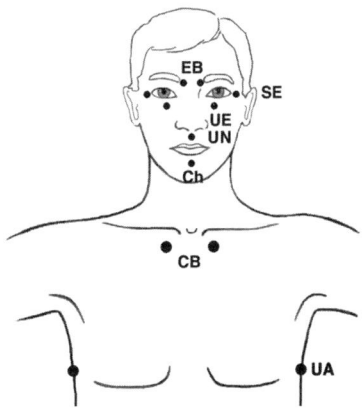

EB, SE, UE, UN, Ch, CB and UA Points

seven to ten times on each point. We call this a "round" of tapping. While tapping, focus on your pain.

EB = Beginning of the EyeBrow

SE = Side of the Eye

UE = Under the Eye

UN = Under the Nose

Ch = Chin

CB = Beginning of the CollarBone

UA = Under the Arm

In EFT, it's important to measure your results frequently, to determine if you're making progress. Again, tune into the painful body location you chose. Using the same scale from 0 to 10, with 0 being no pain and 10 being the worst pain imaginable, rate the level of your pain now. Write down that number. If your pain is at 0, congratulations! You are one of those we call "one-minute wonders." Though some people do experience such quick relief with EFT, it is more common to have some pain still after one round. In that case, we simply tap again.

My pain after my first round of EFT:

No Pain—0 1 2 3 4 5 6 7 8 9 10—Maximum Pain

A Second Helping of EFT

This time, we'll use a slightly different Setup Statement. Most people experience a reduction in pain, so we'll modify the statement accordingly:

> *Even though I still have some pain in _____, I deeply and completely accept myself.*

Say this three times while tapping on the Karate Chop point.

Now tap lightly seven to ten times with two fingertips on each of the EFT points. While tapping, focus on your remaining pain.

When you are finished, again rate your pain level on the 0-to-10 scale. As before, write down that number.

My pain after my second round of EFT:

No Pain—0 1 2 3 4 5 6 7 8 9 10—Maximum Pain

A Final Round of EFT

You might still have some remaining pain, so for good measure, let's try EFT again.

> *Even though I still have some remaining pain in _____, I deeply and completely accept myself.*

Say this three times while tapping on the Karate Chop point.

Now tap lightly seven to ten times with two fingertips on each of the other EFT points. While tapping, focus on your remaining pain.

Measure Your Results

Let's measure the results a final time to see how EFT helped your pain level. Tune in again to the body location you focused on while tapping. How is your pain now on the 0-to-10 scale?

My pain after my third round of EFT:

No Pain—0 1 2 3 4 5 6 7 8 9 10—Maximum Pain

Most people experience a reduction in their pain with this simple exercise. If you did, you have just had a clear demonstration of how effective EFT is in reducing pain. Did you believe, half an hour ago, that you could reduce your pain by any amount, all by yourself, within minutes, using a simple tool like EFT? EFT can also be effective with many of the other symptoms of fibromyalgia, chronic fatigue syndrome, Lyme, and other autoimmune conditions.

If you didn't experience a reduction in your pain level, read on. In the chapters that follow, you will get further tips on tapping, learn about factors that can interfere with tapping, and receive guidance on how to apply EFT in the most successful way for you.

The following story by Sarah Marshall moved me deeply. You will probably identify with her symptoms, and the combination of anxiety, desperation, and searching she went through on her journey to find healing.

Success Story: Fully Recovered from CFS

By Sarah L. Marshall, BSc (Hons)

I struggled with chronic fatigue for six years and was unable to work for over four of those years. At the age of twenty-seven, I was having days of unrelenting dizziness, I felt as though I had a flu that wasn't getting better, I couldn't concentrate (even just making a cup of tea seemed a challenge at times), and I didn't have the energy to do anything more than sit around waiting for it to pass. I felt as though a plug had been pulled and all of my energy with it. It didn't feel like normal tiredness and I was frightened. All my doctor had to say was that I couldn't expect to have the energy I had as a seventeen-year-old. I desperately needed answers or at least my doctor's support and this is what she offered me. I remember thinking…actually I can't repeat exactly what I thought as it involved a number of strong phrases! But I do remember thinking, "I might believe you if I was eighty-seven, not twenty-seven!"

This was one of numerous events that triggered a strong anxiety, which I experienced for the majority of my illness. I was anxious about the confusing symptoms, the inability of my doctors to diagnose what was wrong, my inability to convince some of the medical doctors I consulted that I was ill at all. I felt helpless and panicked about the unrelenting fatigue and the fact that for a number of years whatever I did just seemed to make it worse.

Another event that stuck clearly in my mind was just after I had been diagnosed with CFS, which took over a year. I remember an initial feeling of relief. At last, I had found what was actually wrong with me. At that time, I knew little about the illness. The specialist who delivered the diagnosis didn't tell me how to approach recovery, apart from the suggestion of learning how to breathe properly. But after all that time of searching for an answer, I felt as though I was getting somewhere at last. Afterward, I went back to the flat I shared with friends. They could see from the relief on my face that the appointment had gone well.

I shared what the specialist had said. One of my flat mates revealed that she had a colleague with the same condition. Eager to know more, I asked her for details and she said that her colleague was doing really well, in fact she was now up to a couple of hours of work after five years of illness. I was floored that a couple of hours of work daily might be all I could hope for in five years. This triggered a panic attack that lasted almost a day.

Unfortunately, I didn't discover EFT until I was improving using other methods. Where EFT came into its own for me was to ensure that the progress I had finally started making was sustainable. In hindsight, I can see that anxiety and panic were the two main factors perpetuating many of my symptoms, such as dizziness, breathlessness, and visual disturbances. These, for me, were more disabling than the more physical symptoms such as fatigue and joint and muscle pain. I was anxious about my symptoms, the fact I didn't know what was causing them. All I knew was that if I did anything more than ten to fifteen minutes of physical or cognitive activity, I would feel worse. I had fears about the future, and fears about being able to cope if I lost my financial support. I became frightened of life and my ability to cope with it. I'd also lost all trust in my body and its ability to be healthy.

I started using EFT on my fears regarding my symptoms. This helped reduce my anxiety level. As I worked through the emotional component of the issue, my symptoms began to subside. I worked

About Fibromyalgia and Chronic Fatigue 17

on my future fears, related to "doing too much" or overdoing it. I did this by tapping on the emotional charge I felt around past times when I had engaged in a physical activity and felt worse afterward. I then moved onto what I feared would happen in the future and what impact it would have, again always tracing it back to the earliest event of when I had experienced each specific fear. This again helped with the anxiety I felt around trying something again in the future. Slowly, I found I was able to do more.

I then started working through past contributing factors, going back to childhood and all the memories that had upheld my beliefs and behavior around control, the perceived control I felt others had over my life, my lack of potency around being able to change my situation, and the two memories I described around diagnosis and possible prognosis.

I also was led back to what was going on around the time when my illness began and the events of the preceding year. I was working a high-pressure job as an IT programmer. The majority of our programming was on a live system; one wrong keystroke could have dramatic implications for the system and the end-users. We could bring down the system dependent on the programs we were updating. The pressure, the fact that I wasn't looking after myself, and the low self-esteem I had suffered from since being a very shy child all impacted my health and made me susceptible to illness.

I used EFT on each issue and tapped through each event that upheld an aspect of the issue. It wasn't easy. Nor was it quick—no one-minute wonders for me. But by being consistent, I started to chip away at the issues and slowly collapse them to a point where I was free of the constant anxiety I had felt about my symptoms and my body's abilities, especially regarding activity. This, for me, was key in moving forward and regaining my health. It enabled me to take the pressure off my system. For the first time in years, I started to relax. This enabled my body to upregulate the parasympathetic nervous system and start to repair and restore my body. I had already started to do this with other techniques, but the anxiety triggered by past experiences was always a blocking factor.

I haven't cleared all of the issues that culminated in CFS, but I worked through and collapsed them enough to be able to restore myself to full health. I am now fully recovered and have been for about seven years. EFT is the technique that ensured I fully overcame the condition.

I do continue with self-work to clear what is left, not because I fear becoming ill again—I can say, hand on heart, that I will never again experience ME (myalgic encephalomyelitis, the British term for CFS)—but because I feel it is important, for me personally and as part of being a practitioner. After recovering, I trained in EFT so I could help others with this condition.

※ ※ ※

Imagine yourself having the same healing experience as Sarah. Her story of success could be your story. Why not? You'll hear many such stories throughout this book, and find more on the EFTuniverse.com website. Even people who'd had symptoms for many years, and had no expectation that they could get better, have experienced positive results with EFT. We'll share their stories with you frequently in the pages to come, to fill your mind with the possibility of healing, and inspire you to persevere with EFT through any setbacks you encounter. Sarah, in fact, went on to train as an EFT practitioner, and you will find several stories of the help she offered other sufferers on the EFTuniverse.com site.

Now let's learn more about fibromyalgia, chronic fatigue, and similar challenging health conditions.

Similarities Between Health Conditions

The reason that this book covers fibromyalgia and chronic fatigue, as well as frequently mentioning Lyme disease and other autoimmune conditions, becomes obvious when we examine the similarities between the main symptoms of these disorders. While the following symptoms are drawn from medical descriptions of fibromyalgia and chronic fatigue, if you're suffering from other autoimmune diseases, you're likely to see similarities with your condition. The similarity of symptoms is one reason why Lyme disease is often misdiagnosed as chronic fatigue or fibromyalgia, and vice versa, as well as a variety of other misdiagnoses. Don't worry too much about your diagnosis when using this book, because EFT may be able to help regardless of your particular collection of symptoms.

Symptoms of Fibromyalgia	Symptoms of CFS
Extreme fatigue Pain all over Morning stiffness Muscle knots, cramping, weakness Sleep problems Brain fog Memory and concentration problems Headaches/migraines Irritable bowel/digestive disorders Depression Anxiety Blurred vision Balance problems Fever Reduced ability to exercise Hypersensitivity to cold and heat Sun sensitivity Rash, hives, itchy/burning skin Numbness and tingling in hands and feet	Extreme fatigue Unexplained muscle pain Joint pain without swelling or redness Sleep problems Brain fog Memory and concentration problems Headaches Irritable bowel/digestive disorders Depression Anxiety, panic attacks Irritability, mood swings Visual disturbances Balance problems or fainting Fever or low temperature Increased fatigue and sickness for more than 24 hours after physical or mental exercise Allergies or sensitivities to foods, odors, chemicals, medications, or noise Numbness, tingling, or burning sensations in the face, hands, or feet Chills and night sweats Sore throat Tender lymph nodes

About Fibromyalgia and Chronic Fatigue

With the symptoms being so nearly identical, it is often difficult, if not impossible, to distinguish one disorder from the other. In fact, many patients receive a dual diagnosis. So whether you have been told you have fibromyalgia, CFS, both, Lyme, an autoimmune disease, or you're not sure what you have, you can use EFT to reduce or eliminate your symptoms and greatly improve your physical, emotional, and mental health. All of the procedures and most of the discussions in this book apply equally to fibromyalgia, CFS, and similar conditions, even when only fibromyalgia is mentioned. For the sake of brevity, rather than repeating the names of all disorders in every instance, the book focuses on fibromyalgia. Please use it as shorthand for any similar symptoms you might have.

Here are some other similarities between fibromyalgia and CFS. An estimated five million Americans suffer from fibromyalgia; four million suffer from CFS (some experts cite the numbers for both as much higher and there is likely overlap in those affected, given dual diagnoses). Both disorders afflict vastly more women than men. Onset of both health conditions is most common in young adulthood through middle age. The cause of fibromyalgia? Unknown. The cause of CFS? Unknown. The cause of most autoimmune disease? Unknown. The good news is that you don't need to know the cause of your illness in order to reduce your symptoms with EFT!

A Self-Test for Fibromyalgia

What is your fibromyalgia score? Take this test to find out.

1. Widespread Pain Index (WPI)

Put a check next to the areas where you have had pain over the last week. Add up your checkmarks. Your score will be between 0 and 19.

___ Shoulder area, left

___ Shoulder area, right

___ Upper arm, left

___ Upper arm, right

___ Lower arm, left

___ Lower arm, right

___ Hip/buttock area, left

___ Hip/buttock area, right

___ Upper leg, left

___ Upper leg, right

___ Lower leg, left

___ Lower leg, right

___ Jaw, left

___ Jaw, right

___ Chest

___ Abdomen

___ Upper back

___ Lower back

___ Neck

___ **My Total WPI Score**

2. Symptom Severity (SS) Scale Score

A. Rate the level of severity of your symptoms in the past week in each of the following three areas, using 0 for no problem; 1 for slight or mild problems, generally mild or intermittent; 2 for moderate, considerable problems, often present and/or at a moderate level; and 3 for severe: pervasive, continuous, life-disturbing problems:

___ Fatigue

___ Waking unrefreshed

___ Cognitive symptoms

___ **My Total Score for Part A** (add your three numbers)

B. ___ How extensive are your symptoms in general? Enter a number in the blank, using 0 for no symptoms, 1 for a few symptoms, 2 for a moderate number of symptoms, and 3 for a great deal of symptoms. You may want to consult the following list of fibromyalgia symptoms: muscle pain, muscle weakness, fatigue or tiredness, irritable bowel syndrome, difficulty thinking or remembering, headache, numbness or tingling, dizziness, insomnia, depression, nervousness, frequent urination, painful urination, bladder spasm, abdominal pain or cramps, constipation, diarrhea, nausea, vomiting, heartburn, oral ulcers, dry mouth, loss of or change in taste, loss of appetite, chest pain, fever, blurred vision, dry eyes, tinnitus, hearing problems, seizures, shortness of breath, wheezing, Raynaud's, itching, hives or welts, rash, sun sensitivity, easy bruising, hair loss.

___ **My Score for Part B**

C. To get your SS scale score, add **A** (your ratings of the severity of the three symptoms—fatigue, waking unrefreshed, cognitive symptoms) and **B** (the extent of your symptoms). Your final score will be between 0 and 12.

___ **My Total SS Score**

For a diagnosis of fibromyalgia, according to proposed new criteria, the following three conditions must be present:

- WPI of 7 or more, and SS scale score of 5 or more, or WPI of 3–6 and SS scale score of 9 or more.
- Your symptoms have been at about this level for at least three months.
- You don't have any other disorder that could be the source of your pain.

Source: adapted from the new diagnostic criteria developed by Frederick Wolfe, MD, et al. "The American College of Rheumatology Preliminary Diagnostic Criteria for Fibromyalgia and Measurement of Symptom Severity." *Arthritis Care and Research* 62:5 (May 2010); 600–610.

Self-Test for Fibromyalgia

It's a good idea to establish a baseline of your illness before you do any further tapping on your symptoms. That way, when you've finished the book, you can compare just how much EFT has helped you. It often happens that people forget how bad they felt before they began tapping (this is called the "apex effect," which you'll read about in chapter 2). You may find it hard to imagine ever forgetting how terrible you feel at this moment or yesterday or the day before, but trust me, it's happened to a lot of people with fibromyalgia who found relief through EFT. May you be one of them!

Take the Self-test for Fibromyalgia to assess the severity of your illness, then again after using EFT for a few weeks, or completing the 12-week program for Fibromyalgia and Chronic Fatigue at EFTuniverse.com. (Save your results so you can compare them later.) If you would rather not do the full self-test, you can simply rate the state of your health by assigning it a number on a scale of 0 to 10, where 0 is fully bedridden and 10 is fully functioning.

The Case for EFT

If you need more persuading to try EFT on your illness, consider the research. In a study of eighty-six women, aged twenty to sixty-five, who had been diagnosed with fibromyalgia less than five years before and had been on sick leave for three or more months, researcher Gunilla Brattberg, MD, of Lund University and Uppsala University in Sweden, compared the effects of self-administered EFT (treatment group) with no treatment (a wait-listed control group) on pain perception, acceptance and coping ability, and health-related quality of life. The treatment group performed EFT daily for eight weeks. The improvements in the EFT group were statistically significant in comparison to the control group for variables of pain, anxiety, depression, vitality, social function, mental health, performance problems involving work or other activities due to physical and/or emotional reasons, and symptoms of stress. Further, "pain catastrophizing measures" (e.g., rumination, magnification, and helplessness) went down significantly while activity levels went up significantly in the EFT group versus the non-treatment group. The number needed to treat (NNT) regarding recovering from anxiety was 3. The NNT for depression was 4.

The concept of NNT is important to know about if you are taking medication. NNT means the number of people you have to give the treatment or drug to in order for one person to benefit. For example, the NNT of 3 for anxiety in Dr. Brattberg's study meant that three people had to do EFT before one person benefitted. The higher the NNT number is, the poorer the returns from the treatment. To put Dr. Brattberg's numbers in perspective, Lipitor, a drug widely prescribed to lower cholesterol, and the best-selling drug in the United States, has an NNT of 100. Despite the fact that one hundred people need to be treated before one benefits, this drug is accepted as the treatment of choice. The most optimal treatment would have an NNT of 1, meaning that each person receiving the treatment benefits from it. Compare these results: the top-selling drug in the United States, with an NNT of 100; a safe, self-applied method like EFT with an NNT of 3 to 4. As more research on EFT is conducted, with refined tapping guidance for subjects, we may see even better NNTs than the already impressive results shown in Dr. Brattberg's study.

Aside from the NNT, there is another parameter you might want to consider regarding medications you're taking. The NNT does not reflect negative side effects. For that, we turn to the NNH, which stands for the "number needed to harm." With the NNH, the lower number is the bad one; that is, an NNH of 5 means that it only takes five people taking it for one person to experience harmful effects. Pregabalin (brand name Lyrica), an anti-seizure medication touted for use in reducing the pain of fibromyalgia, has an NNT of 5, which might not be so bad, but its NNH is reportedly close to 1. That means that nearly every person taking it will experience harmful effects. Xanax, an antianxiety drug often prescribed for fibromyalgia patients, has an NNT of 6 (six people treated before one benefits) and an NNH of 3 (three people treated, one harmed). You might want to research the NNTs and NNHs of medications you are taking. Just because a drug is widely used doesn't mean it is effective or safe.

I am not saying that you should modify the use of any medication you might be taking. You should always consult with your physician when considering any change to your medication. What I am stressing is the importance of getting the best of all worlds, conventional and alterna-

About Fibromyalgia and Chronic Fatigue

tive. It's just always a good idea to educate yourself about anything that might affect your health.

To that end, it's important for you to know that EFT has no harmful side effects. The NNH is too high to count, if it exists at all. This book has plenty of information about EFT, as well as success stories from people who have used EFT for their fibromyalgia and chronic fatigue with good results. And there's plenty more information at www.EFTuniverse.com if you'd like to learn more about the technique and read other accounts by people who successfully resolved a range of ailments using EFT. More research results on the effectiveness of EFT are also available there. Further studies investigating the application of this relatively new technique to a variety of physical and psychological problems are in progress. I myself am currently conducting a large randomized controlled study, which is the highest standard in scientific research, to compare the results of EFT with cognitive behavior therapy (used to manage fibromyalgic symptoms) in the treatment of fibromyalgia. Stay tuned!

Before we move on to the next chapter, which teaches you the very simple EFT protocol called the Basic Recipe, I'd like to share with you one more inspiring story of the progress made by someone suffering from these terrible symptoms. This story comes from certified EFT practitioner Stephen Carter. As is the case with "Susan," the names and identifying details of all clients described in this book have been changed to protect their privacy.

Success Story: Rapid Progress with Fibromyalgia, Depression, and Anxiety

By Stephen Carter, MA, Certified EFT Int-1 Practitioner

Susan, twenty-four, sought my help for pain caused by fibromyalgia and Lyme disease, and for anxiety and depression. She had been diagnosed with Lyme disease four years ago and with fibromyalgia two years ago. She had been under professional care for anxiety and depression but was not taking medication for those conditions when she consulted me.

When she described her current physical symptoms, she mentioned that her breathing felt labored. As a starting point for her to experience EFT, we tapped to increase her breathing capacity.

I explained the steps for evaluating her felt sense of breathing restriction. We used the 0-to-10 scale, with 10 being what she believed was her maximum breathing potential. After three deep breaths and then the evaluation breath, she rated her current breathing at a 7 in comparison to what she believed was possible.

We used the shortcut tapping sequence and added the thumb point (lung meridian) with the Setup affirmations:

"Even though I have this restricted breathing at about a 7 give or take, I deeply and completely accept myself."

"Even though I have this restriction of breath, I choose to accept myself completely breathing limitation and all."

"Even with this breathing limitation rated at about a 7 give or take, I accept myself as a kind, caring and loving person."

After the Setup affirmations, we tapped through the points, using the Reminder Phrases:

"This breath restriction."
"This breathing restriction."
"This restriction."

We ended at the crown point with: *"I choose to release this breathing restriction."*

Upon completion of the breathing restriction sequence, I again asked Susan to test her breathing and compare it to what she believed was possible. She reported that it "might be a little better" and rated it as "maybe a 7 and a half." After further work, Susan reported it was at least a 9 and maybe close to 10. She added that she felt calm and relaxed.

We then turned our attention to her felt sense of physical pain. She reported that pain was present virtually every waking moment, but the intensity rose and fell depending on the time of day, weather conditions, and her level of stress. She reported a general overall current sense of joint pain at a 4. We tapped using the shortcut sequence and Setup affirmations that included:

"Even though I have this joint pain at a 4 level give or take..."

"Even though this constant pain is annoying and tiresome..."

"Even though I have this joint pain in my knees, my shoulders, and my wrists..."

Her Reminder Phrases included:

"This pain."

"This annoying pain."

"This joint pain."

We ended at the crown point with: *"I choose to release this joint pain now."*

After asking her to take a deep breath and release, I asked her to estimate her current joint pain. She replied, "About a 2. It's much less in my knees, but my shoulders still hurt, but not as much."

I asked if one shoulder felt more painful. She replied the pain was more noticeable in her right shoulder compared to her left. We again tapped, using the Setup affirmations:

"Even though I still have some of this joint pain..."

"Even though there is some of this joint pain remaining in my shoulders, particularly in the joint of my right shoulder..."

"Even though there is some pain remaining..."

The Reminder Phrases included:

"This remaining joint pain."
"This joint pain that remains."
"This remaining pain."

Ending at the crown point, she said, *"I choose to release this remaining joint pain."*

At the conclusion of the second round, I asked Susan to rate her joint pain level again. She reported that it was almost gone, "maybe a half."

We ended with a floor-to-ceiling eye roll [covered in *The EFT Manual*] that brought the pain rating to zero. She reported that not only was the pain gone, but also she felt deeply relaxed and calm, adding, "I really feel good. This is great!"

At the conclusion of our first session, Susan was pain free, with no depression or anxiety. I emphasized to her the importance of daily application of EFT for all physical and emotional issues.

Susan stayed in touch over the following two months and reported rapid progress in pain relief and emotional well-being. She is again able to work and continues to use EFT daily.

※ ※ ※

Can you imagine your pain, depression, and anxiety going away after just one session of EFT, like Susan's did? That probably seems too good to be true. Like Sarah, who told us she had no "one-minute wonders," your progress may be slow. Yet many who try EFT report an almost-bewildering disappearance of their symptoms. Please keep your mind open to the possibility that you could get better, like Susan and Sarah did, and that your improvement might be more rapid than you dare believe.

2

How to Do EFT: The Basic Recipe

Over the past decade, EFT has been the focus of a great deal of research. This has resulted in more than twenty clinical trials, in which EFT has been demonstrated to reduce a wide variety of symptoms. These include pain, skin rashes, fibromyalgia, depression, anxiety, and posttraumatic stress disorder (PTSD). Most of these studies have used the standardized form of EFT found in *The EFT Manual*. In this chapter, my goal is to show you how to unlock EFTs healing benefits from whatever physical or psychological problems you're facing. I have a passionate interest in relieving human suffering. When you study EFT, you quickly realize how much suffering can be alleviated with the help of this extraordinary healing tool. I'd like to place the full power of that tool in your hands, so that you can live the happiest, healthiest, and most abundant life possible.

If you go on YouTube or do a Google search, you will find thousands of websites and videos about EFT. The quality of the EFT information you'll find through these sources varies widely, however. Certified practitioners trained in EFT provide a small portion of the information. Most of it consists of personal testimonials by untrained enthusiasts. It's great that EFT works to some degree for virtually anyone. To get the most out of EFT and unlock its full potential, however, it's essential that you learn the form of EFT that's been proven in so many clinical trials. We call this Clinical EFT.

Every year in EFT Universe workshops, we get many people who tell us variations of the same story: "I saw a video on YouTube, tapped along, and got amazing results the first few times. Then it seemed to stop working." The reason for this is that a superficial application of EFT can indeed work wonders. To unleash the full power of EFT, however, requires learning the standardized form we call Clinical EFT, which has been validated, over and over again, by high-quality research, and is taught systematically, step by step, by top experts, in EFT workshops.

Why is EFT able to affect so many problems, both psychological and physical? The reason for its effectiveness is that it reduces stress, and stress is a component of many problems. In EFT research on pain, for instance, we find that pain decreases by an average of 68 percent with EFT. That's a two-thirds drop, and seems very impressive. Now ask yourself, if EFT can produce a two-thirds drop in pain, why can't it produce a 100 percent drop? I pondered this question myself, and I asked many therapists and doctors for their theories as to why this might be so.

The consensus is that the two-thirds of pain reduced by EFT is due largely to emotional causes, while the remaining one-third of the pain has a physical derivation. A man I'll call "John" volunteered for a demonstration at an EFT introductory evening at which I presented. He was on crutches, and told us he had a broken leg as a result of a car accident. On a scale of 0 to 10, with 0 being no pain, and 10 being maximum pain, he rated his pain as an 8. The accident had occurred two weeks earlier. My logical scientific brain didn't think EFT would work for John, because his pain was purely physical. I tapped with him anyway. At the end of our session, which lasted less than 15 minutes, his pain was down to a 2. I hadn't tapped on the actual pain with John at all, but rather on all the emotional components of the auto accident.

There were many such components. His wife had urged him to drive to an event, but he didn't want to go. He had resentment toward his wife. That's emotional. He was angry at the driver of the other car. That's emotional. He was mad at himself for abandoning his own needs by driving to an event he didn't want to attend. That's emotional. He was upset that now, as an adult, he was reenacting the abandonment he experienced by his mother when he was a child. That's emotional. He was still hurt by an incident that occurred when he was five years old, when his mother was supposed to pick him up from a friend's birthday party and forgot because she was socializing with her friends and drinking. That's emotional.

Do you see the pattern here? We're working on a host of problems that are emotional, yet interwoven with the pain. The physical pain is overlaid with a matrix of emotional issues, like self-neglect, abandonment, anger, and frustration, which are part of the entire fabric of John's life.

The story has a happy ending. After we'd tapped on each of these emotional components of John's pain, the physical pain in his broken leg went down to a 2. That pain rating revealed the extent of the physical component of John's problem. It was a 2. The other six points were emotional.

The same is true for the person who's afraid of public speaking, who has a spider phobia, who's suffering from a physical ailment, who's feeling trapped in his job, who's unhappy with her husband, who's in conflict with those around him. All of these problems have a large component of unfinished emotional business from the past. When you neutralize the underlying emotional issues with EFT, what remains is the real problem, which is often far smaller than you imagine.

Though I present at few conferences nowadays because of other demands on my time, I used to present at about thirty medical and psychological conferences each year, speaking about research and teaching EFT. I presented to thousands of medical professionals during that period. One of my favorite sayings was "Don't medicalize emotional problems. And don't emotionalize medical problems." When I would say this to a roomful of physicians, they would nod their heads in unison. The medical profession as a whole is very aware of the emotional component of disease.

How to Do EFT: The Basic Recipe

If you have a real medical problem, you need good medical care. No ifs, ands, or buts. If you have an emotional problem, you need EFT. Most problems are a mixture of both. That's why I urge you to work on the emotional component with EFT and other safe and noninvasive behavioral methods, and to get the best possible medical care for the physical component of your problem. Talk to your doctor about this; virtually every physician will be supportive of you bolstering your medical treatment with emotional catharsis.

When you feel better emotionally, a host of positive changes also occur in your energy system. When you feel worse, your energy system follows. Several researchers have hooked people up to electroencephalographs (EEGs), and taken EEG readings of the electrical energy in their brains before and after EFT. These studies show that when subjects are asked to recall a traumatic event, their patterns of brain-wave activity change. The brain-wave frequencies associated with stress, and activation of the fight-or-flight response, dominate their EEG readings. After successful treatment, the brain waves shown on their EEG readings are those that characterize relaxation.

Other research has shown similar results from acupuncture. The theory behind acupuncture is that our body's energy flows in twelve channels called meridians. When that energy is blocked, physical or psychological distress occurs. The use of acupuncture needles, or acupressure with the fingertips, is believed to release those energy blocks. EFT has you tap with your fingertips on the end points of those meridians; that's why it's sometimes called "emotional acupuncture." When your energy is balanced and flowing, whether it's the brain-wave energy picked up by the EEG or the meridian energy described in acupuncture, you feel better. That's another reason why EFT works well for many different kinds of problem.

EFT is rooted in sound science, and this chapter is devoted to showing you how to do Clinical EFT yourself. It will introduce you to the basic concepts that amplify the power of EFT, and steer you clear of the most common pitfalls that prevent people from making progress with EFT. The basics of EFT are easy to use and quick to learn. We call this EFT's "Basic Recipe." The second half of this chapter shows you how to apply the Basic Recipe for maximum effect. It introduces you to all of the concepts key to Clinical EFT.

Testing

EFT doesn't just hope to be effective. We test our results constantly, to determine if the course we're taking is truly making us feel better. The basic scale we use for testing was developed by a famous psychiatrist called Joseph Wolpe in the 1950s, and measures our degree of discomfort on a scale of 0 through 10. Zero indicates no discomfort, and 10 is the maximum possible distress. This scale works equally well for psychological problems such as anxiety and physical problems such as pain.

How to Do EFT: The Basic Recipe

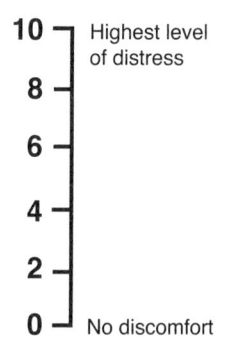

```
10 ─┐  Highest level
     │  of distress
 8 ─┤
 6 ─┤
 4 ─┤
 2 ─┤
 0 ─┘  No discomfort
```

SUD scale (intensity meter)

Dr. Wolpe called this rating SUD or Subjective Units of Disturbance. It's also sometimes called Subjective Units of Distress. You feel your problem, and give it a number on the SUD scale. It's vital to rate your SUD level as it is *right now*, not imagine what it might have been at the time in the past when the traumatic event occurred. If you can't quickly identify a number, just take your best guess, and go from there.

I recommend you write down your initial SUD number. It's also worth noting *where in your body* the information on your SUD level is coming from. If you're working on a physical pain such as a headache, where in your head is the ache centered? If you're working on a traumatic emotional event, perhaps a car accident, where in your body is your reference point for your emotional distress? Do you feel it in your belly, your heart, your forehead? Write down the location on which your SUD is based.

A variation of the numeric scale is a visual scale. For example, if you're working with a child who does not yet know how to count, you can ask the child to spread his or her hands apart to indicate how big the problem is. Wide-open arms means big, and hands close together means small.

Whatever means you use to test, each round of EFT tapping usually begins with this type of assessment of the size of the problem. This allows us to determine whether or not our approach is working. After we've tested and written down our SUD level and body location, we move on to EFTs Basic Recipe. It has this name to indicate that EFT consists of certain ingredients, and if you want to be successful, you need to include them, just the way you need to include all the ingredients in a recipe for chocolate chip cookies if you want your end product to be tasty.

Many years ago I published a book by Wally Amos. Wally is better known as "Famous Amos" for his brand of chocolate chip cookies. One day I asked Wally, "Where did you get your recipe?" I thought he was going to tell me how he'd experimented with hundreds of variations to find the best possible combination of ingredients. I imagined Wally like Thomas Edison in his laboratory, obsessively combining pinches of this and smidgeons of that, year after year, in order to perfect the flavor of his cookies, the way Edison tried thousands of combinations before discovering the incandescent light bulb.

Wally's offhand response was, "I used the recipe on the back of a pack of Toll House chocolate chips." Toll House is one of the most popular brands, selling millions of packages each year, and the simple recipe is available to everyone. I was astonished, and laughed at how different the reality was from my imaginary picture of Wally as Edison. Yet the message is simple: Don't reinvent the wheel. If it works, it works. Toll House is so popular because their recipe works. Clinical EFT produces such good results because the Basic Recipe works. While a master chef might be experienced enough to produce exquisite variations, a beginner can bake excellent cookies, and get consistently great results, just by following the basic recipe. This chapter is designed to provide you with that simple yet reliable level of knowledge.

EFTs Basic Recipe omits a procedure that was part of the earliest forms of EFT, called the 9 Gamut Procedure. Though the 9 Gamut Procedure has great value for certain conditions, it isn't always necessary, so we leave it out. The version of EFT that includes it is called the Full Basic Recipe (see chapter 3).

The Setup Statement

The Setup Statement systematically "sets up" the problem you want to work on. Think about arranging dominoes in a line in the game of creating a chain reaction. Before you start the game, you set them up. The object of the game is to knock them down, just the way EFT expects to knock down your SUD level, but to start with, you set up the pieces of the problem.

The Setup Statement has its roots in two schools of psychology. One is called cognitive therapy, and the other is called exposure therapy. Cognitive therapy considers the large realm of your cognitions—your thoughts, beliefs, ways of relating to others, and the mental frames through which you perceive the world and your experiences.

Exposure therapy is a successful branch of psychotherapy that vividly exposes you to your negative experiences. Rather than avoiding them, you're confronted by them, with the goal of breaking your conditioned fear response to the event.

We won't go deeper into these two forms of therapy now, but you'll later see how EFT's Setup Statement draws from cognitive and exposure approaches to form a powerful combination with acupressure or tapping.

Psychological Reversal

The term Psychological Reversal is taken from energy therapies. It refers to the concept that when your energies are blocked or reversed, you develop symptoms. If you put the batteries into a flashlight backward, with the positive end where the negative should be, the light won't shine. The human body also has a polarity (see illustration). A reversal of normal polarity will block the flow of energy through the body. In acupuncture, the goal of treatment is to remove obstructions, and to allow the free flow of energy through the twelve meridians. If reversal occurs, it impedes the healing process.

How to Do EFT: The Basic Recipe

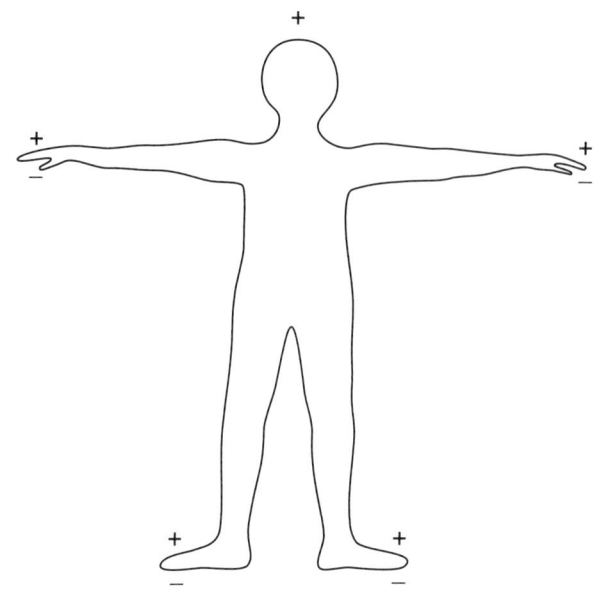

The human body's electrical polarity (adapted from *ACEP Certification Program Manual,* 2006)

The way Psychological Reversal shows up in EFT and other energy therapies is as a failure to make progress in resolving the problem. It's especially prevalent in chronic diseases, addictions, and conditions that resist healing. If you run into a person who's desperate to recover, yet who has had no success even with a wide variety of different therapies, the chances are good that you're dealing with Psychological Reversal. One of the first steps of EFTs Basic Recipe is to correct for Psychological Reversal. It only takes a few seconds, so we include this step whether or not Psychological Reversal is present.

EFTs Setup includes stating an affirmation with those elements drawn from cognitive and exposure therapies, while at the same time correcting for Psychological Reversal.

Affirmation

The exposure part of the Setup Statement involves remembering the problem. You expose your mind repeatedly to the memory of the trauma. This is the opposite of what we normally do; we usually want an emotional trauma to fade away. We might engage in behaviors like dissociation or avoidance so that we don't have to deal with unpleasant memories.

As you gain confidence with EFT, you'll find yourself becoming fearless when it comes to exposure. You'll discover you don't have to remain afraid of old traumatic memories; you have a tool that allows you to reduce their emotional intensity in minutes or even seconds. The usual pattern of running away from a problem is reversed. You feel confident running toward it, knowing that you'll quickly feel better.

The EFT Setup Statement is this: *Even though I have (name of problem), I deeply and completely accept myself.*

You insert the name of the problem in the exposure half of the Setup Statement. Examples might be:

Even though I had that dreadful car crash, I deeply and completely accept myself.

Even though I have this migraine headache, I deeply and completely accept myself.

How to Do EFT: The Basic Recipe   45

Even though I have this fear of heights, I deeply and completely accept myself.

Even though I have this pain in my knees, I deeply and completely accept myself.

Even though I had my buddy die in my arms in Iraq, I deeply and completely accept myself.

Even though I have this huge craving for whiskey, I deeply and completely accept myself.

Even though I have this fear of spiders, I deeply and completely accept myself.

Even though I have this urge to eat another cookie, I deeply and completely accept myself.

The list of variations is infinite. You can use this Setup Statement for anything that bothers you.

While exposure is represented by the first half of the Setup Statement, before the comma, cognitive work is done by the second half of the statement, the part that deals with self-acceptance. EFT doesn't try to induce you to positive thinking. You don't tell yourself that things will get better, or that you'll improve. You simply express the intention of accepting yourself just the way you are. You accept reality. Gestalt therapist Byron Katie wrote a book entitled *Loving What Is,* and that's exactly what EFT recommends you do.

The Serenity Prayer uses the same formula of acceptance, with the words, "God grant me the serenity to accept the things I cannot change; courage to change the things I can; and wisdom to know the difference." With EFT you don't try and think positively. You don't try and change your attitude or circumstances; you simply affirm that you accept them. This cognitive frame of accepting what is opens the path to change in a profound way. It's also quite difficult to do this in our culture, which bombards us with positive thinking. Positive thinking actually gets in the way of healing in many cases, while acceptance provides us with a reality-based starting point congruent with our experience. The great twentieth-century therapist Carl Rogers, who introduced client-centered therapy, said that the paradox of transformation is that change begins by accepting conditions exactly the way they are.

I recommend that you use the Setup Statement in exactly this way at first, but as you gain confidence, you can experiment with different variations. The only requirement is that you include both a self-acceptance statement and exposure to the problem. For instance, you can invert the two halves of the formula, and put cognitive self-acceptance first, followed by exposure. Here are some examples:

I accept myself fully and completely, even with this miserable headache.

I deeply love myself, even though I have nightmares from that terrible car crash.

I hold myself in high esteem, even though I feel such pain from my divorce.

When you're doing EFT with children, you don't need an elaborate Setup Statement. You can have children use very simple self-acceptance phrases, like "I'm okay" or "I'm a great kid." Such a Setup Statement might look like this:

Even though Johnny hit me, I'm okay.

The teacher was mean to me, but I'm still an amazing kid.

You'll be surprised how quickly children respond to EFT. Their SUD levels usually drop so fast that adults have a difficult time accepting the shift. Although we haven't yet done the research to discover why children are so receptive to change, my hypothesis is that their behaviors haven't yet been cemented by years of conditioning. They've not yet woven a thick neural grid in their brains through repetitive thinking and behavior, so they can let go of negative emotions fast.

What do you do if your problem is self-acceptance itself? What if you believe you're unacceptable? What if you have low self-esteem, and the words "I deeply and completely accept myself" sound like a lie?

What EFT suggests you do in such a case is say the words anyway, even if you don't believe them. They will usually have some effect, even if at first you have difficulty with them. As you correct for Psychological Reversal in the way I will show you here, you will soon find yourself shifting from unbelief to belief that you are acceptable. You can say the affirmation aloud or silently. It carries more emotional energy if it is said emphatically or loudly, and imagined vividly.

Secondary Gain

While energy therapies use the term "psychological reversal" to indicate energy blocks to healing, there's an equivalent term drawn from psychology. That term is "secondary gain." It refers to the benefits of being sick. "Why would anyone want to be sick?" you might wonder. There are actually many reasons for keeping a mental or physical problem firmly in place.

Consider the case of a veteran with PTSD. He's suffering from flashbacks of scenes from Afghanistan where he witnessed death and suffering. He has nightmares, and never sleeps through the night. He's so disturbed that he cannot hold down a job or keep a relationship intact for long. Why would such a person not want to get better, considering the damage PTSD is doing to his life?

The reason might be that he's getting a disability check each month as a result of his condition. His income is dependent on having PTSD, and if he recovers, his main source of livelihood might disappear with it.

Another reason might be that he was deeply wounded by a divorce many years ago. He lost his house and children in the process. He's fearful of getting into another romantic relationship that is likely to end badly. PTSD gives him a reason to not try.

These are obvious examples of secondary gain. When we work with participants in EFT workshops, we uncover a wide variety of subtle reasons that stand in the way of healing. One woman had been trying to lose weight for five years and had failed at every diet she tried. Her secondary gain turned out to be freedom from unwanted attention by men.

Another woman, this time with fibromyalgia, discovered that her secret benefit from the disease was that she didn't have to visit relatives she didn't like. She had a ready excuse for avoiding social obligations. She also got sympathetic attention from her husband and children for her suffering. If she gave up her painful disease, she might lose a degree of affection from her family and have to resume seeing the relatives she detested.

Just like Psychological Reversal, secondary gain prevents us from making progress on our healing journey. Correcting for these hidden obstacles to success is one of the first elements in EFTs Basic Recipe.

How EFT Corrects for Psychological Reversal

The first tapping point we use in the EFT routine is called the Karate Chop point, because it's located on the fleshy outer portion of the hand, the part used in karate to deliver a blow. EFT has you tap the Karate Chop point with the tips of the other four fingers of the opposite hand

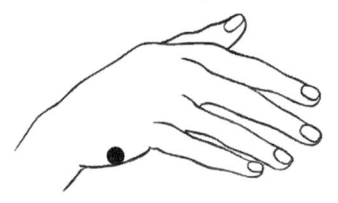

The Karate Chop (KC) Point

Repeat your affirmation emphatically three times while tapping your Karate Chop point. You've now corrected for psychological reversal, and set up your energy system for the next part of EFTs Basic Recipe, the Sequence.

The Sequence

You now tap on meridian end points in sequence. Tap firmly, but not harshly, with the tips of your first two fingers, about seven times on each point. The exact number is not important; it can be a few more or less than seven. You can tap on either the right or left side of your body, with either your dominant or nondominant hand.

First tap on the meridian endpoints found on the face. These are: (1) at the start of the eyebrow, where it joins the bridge of the nose; (2) on the outside edge of the eye socket; (3) on the bony ridge of the eye socket under the pupil; (4) under the nose; and (5) between the lower lip and the chin.

EB, SE, UE, UN and Ch Points

Then tap (6) on one of the collarbone points (see illustration). To locate this point, place a finger in the notch between your collarbones. Move your finger down about an inch and you'll feel a hollow in your breastbone.

How to Do EFT: The Basic Recipe 51

Now move it to the side about an inch and you'll find a deep hollow below your collarbone. You've now located the collarbone acupressure point.

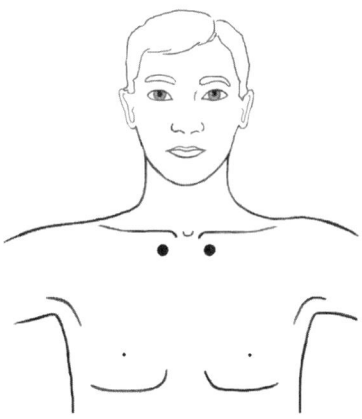

The Collarbone (CB) Points

About four inches below the armpit (for women, this is where a bra strap crosses), you'll find (7) the under the arm point.

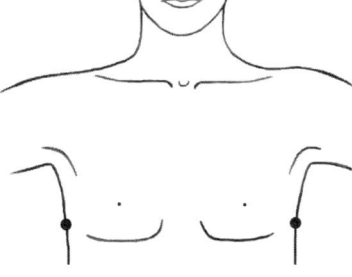

Under the Arm (UA) Points

The Reminder Phrase

Earlier, I emphasized the importance of exposure. Exposure therapy has been the subject of much research, which has shown that prolonged exposure to a problem, when coupled with techniques to calm the body, effectively treats traumatic stress. EFT incorporates exposure in the form of a Reminder Phrase. This is a brief phrase that keeps the problem at the front of your mind while you tap on the acupressure points. It keeps your energy system focused on the specific issue you're working on, rather than jumping to other thoughts and feelings. The aim of the Reminder Phrase is to bring the problem vividly into your experience, even though the emotionally triggering situation might not be present now.

For instance, if you have test anxiety, you use the Reminder Phrase to keep you focused on the fear, even though you aren't actually taking a test right now. That gives EFT an opportunity to shift the pattern in the absence of the real problem. You can also use EFT during an actual situation, such as when you're taking an actual test, but most of the time you're working on troublesome memories. The Reminder Phrase keeps you targeted on the problem. An example of a Reminder Phrase for test anxiety might be *"That test"* or *"The test I have to take tomorrow"* or *"That test I failed."* Other examples of Reminder Phrases are:

The beesting

Dad hit me

Friend doesn't respect me

Lawyer's office

Sister told me I was fat

Car crash

This knee pain

Tap each point while repeating your Reminder Phrase. Then tune in to the problem again, and get a second SUD rating. The chances are good that your SUD score will now be much lower than it was before. These instructions might seem complicated the first time you read them, but you'll soon find you're able to complete a round of EFT tapping from memory in one to two minutes.

Let's now summarize the steps of EFTs Basic Recipe.

1. Assess your SUD level.
2. Insert the name of your problem into the Setup Statement: *"Even though I have (this problem), I deeply and completely accept myself."*
3. Tap continuously on the Karate Chop point while repeating the Setup Statement three times.
4. While repeating the Reminder Phrase, tap about seven times on the other seven points.
5. Test your results with a second SUD rating.

Isn't that simple? You now have a tool that, in just a minute or two, can effectively neutralize the emotional sting of old memories, as well as help you get through bad current situations. After a few rounds of tapping, you'll find you've effortlessly memorized the Basic Recipe, and you'll find yourself using it often in your daily life.

If Your SUD Level Doesn't Come Down to 0

Sometimes a single round of tapping brings your SUD score to 0. Sometimes it only brings it down slightly. Your migraine might have been an 8, and after a round of EFT it's a 4. In these cases, we do EFT again. You can adjust your affirmation to acknowledge that a portion of the problem sill remains, for example, *"Even though I still have some of this migraine, I deeply and completely accept myself."* Hear are some further examples:

Even though I still feel some anger toward my friend for putting me down, I deeply and completely accept myself.

Even though I still have a little twinge of that knee pain, I deeply and completely accept myself.

Even though the beesting still smarts slightly, I deeply and completely accept myself.

Even though I'm still harboring some resentment toward my boss, I deeply and completely accept myself.

Even though I'm still somewhat frustrated with my daughter for breaking her agreement, I deeply and completely accept myself.

Even though I'm still upset when I think of being shipped to Iraq, I deeply and completely accept myself.

Adjust the Reminder Phrase accordingly, as in *"some anger still"* or *"remaining frustration"* or *"bit of pain"* or *"somewhat upset."*

EFT for You and Others

You can do EFT on yourself, as you've experienced during these practice rounds. You can also tap on others. Many therapists, life coaches, and other practitioners offer EFT professionally to clients. Personally I'm far more inclined to have clients tap on themselves during EFT sessions, even during the course of a therapy or coaching session. While the coach can tap on the client, having the client tap on themselves, along with some guidance by the coach, puts the power squarely in the hands of the client. The client is empowered by discovering that they are able to reduce their own emotional distress, and leaves the coaches office with a self-help tool at their fingertips any time they need it. In some jurisdictions, it is illegal or unethical for therapists to touch clients at all, and EFT when done only by the client is still effective in these cases.

The Importance of Targeting Specific Events

During EFT workshops, I sometimes write on the board:

The Three Most Important Things About EFT

Then, under that, I write:

Specific Events

Specific Events

Specific Events

It's my way of driving home the point that a focus on specific events is critical to success in EFT. In order to release old patterns of emotion and behavior, it's vital to identify and correct the specific events that gave rise to those problems. When you hear people say, "I tried EFT and it didn't work," the chances are good that they were tapping on generalities, instead of specifics.

An example of a generality is "self-esteem" or "depression" or "performance problems." These aren't specific events. Beneath these generalities is a collection of specific events. The person with low self-esteem might have been coloring a picture at the age of four when her mother walked in and criticized her for drawing outside the lines. She might have had another experience of a schoolteacher scolding her for playing with her hair during class in second grade, and a third experience of her first boyfriend deciding to ask another girl to the school dance. Together, those specific events contribute to the global pattern of low self-esteem. The way EFT works is that when the emotional trauma of those individual events is resolved, the whole pattern of low self-esteem can shift. If you tap on the big pattern, and omit the specific events, you're likely to have limited success.

When you think about how a big pattern like low self-esteem is established, this makes sense. It's built up out of many single events. Collectively, they form the whole pattern. The big pattern doesn't spring to life fully formed; it's built up gradually out of many similar experiences. The memories engraved in your brain are of individual events; one disappointing or traumatic memory at a time is encoded in your memory bank. When enough similar memories have accumulated, their commonalities combine to create a common theme like "poor self-esteem." Yet the theme originated as a series of specific events, and that's where EFT can be effectively applied.

You don't have to use EFT on every single event that contributed to the global theme. Usually, once a few of the most disturbing memories have lost their emotional impact, the whole pattern disappears. Memories that are similar lose their impact once the most vivid memories have been neutralized with EFT.

Tapping on global issues is the single most common mistake newcomers make with EFT. Using lists of tapping phrases from a website or a book, or tapping on generalities, is far less effective than tuning into the events that contributed to your global problem, and tapping on them. If you hear someone say, "EFT doesn't work," the chances are good they've been tapping globally rather than identifying specific events. Don't make this elementary mistake. List the events, one after the other, that stand out most vividly in your mind when you think about the global problem. Tap on each of them, and you'll usually find the global problem diminishing of its own accord. This is called the "generalization effect," and it's one of the key concepts in EFT.

Tapping on Aspects

EFT breaks traumatic events and other problems into smaller pieces called aspects. The reason for this is that the highest emotional charge is typically found in one small chunk of the event, rather than the entirety of the event. You might need to identify several different aspects, and tap on each of them, before the intensity of the whole event is reduced to a 0.

Here's an example of tapping on aspects, drawn from experience at an EFT workshop I taught. A woman in her late thirties volunteered as a subject. She'd had neck pain and limited range of motion since an automobile accident six years before. She could turn her head to the right most of the way but had only a few degrees of movement to the left. The accident had been a minor one, and why she still suffered six years later was something of a mystery to her.

I asked her to feel where in her body she felt the most intensity when recalling the accident, and she said it was in her upper chest. I then asked her about the first time she'd ever felt that way, and she said it was when she'd been involved in another auto accident at the age of eight. Her sister had been driving the car. We worked on each aspect of the early accident. The two girls had hit another car head on at low speed while driving around a bend on a country road. One emotionally triggering aspect was the moment she realized that a collision was unavoidable, and we tapped till that lost its force. We tapped on the sound of the crash, another aspect. She had been taken to a neighbor's house, bleeding from a cut on her head, and we tapped on that. We tapped on aspect after aspect. Still, her pain level didn't go down much, and her range of motion didn't improve.

Then she gasped and said, "I just remembered. My sister was only fifteen years old. She was underage. That

How to Do EFT: The Basic Recipe

day, I dared her to drive the family car, and we totaled it." Her guilt turned out to be the aspect that held the most emotional charge, and after we tapped on that, her pain disappeared, and she regained full range of motion in her neck. If we'd tapped on the later accident, or failed to uncover all the aspects, we might have thought, "EFT doesn't work."

Aspects can be pains, physical sensations, emotions, images, sounds, tastes, odors, fragments of an event, or beliefs. Make sure you dig deep for all the emotional charge held in each aspect of an event before you move on to the next one. One way of doing this is to check each sensory channel, and ask, "What did you hear/see/taste/touch/smell?" For one person, the burned-rubber smell of skidding tires might be the most terrifying aspect of a car accident. For another, it might be the smell of blood. Yet another person might remember most vividly the sound of the crash or the screams. For another person, the maximum emotional charge might be held in the feeling of terror at the moment of realization that the crash is inevitable. The pain itself might be an aspect. Guilt, or any other emotion, can be an aspect. For traumatic events, it's necessary to tap on each aspect.

Thorough exploration of all the aspects will usually yield a complete neutralization of the memory. If there's still some emotional charge left, the chances are good that you've missed an aspect, so go back and find out what shards of trauma might still be stuck in place.

Finding Core Issues

One of my favorite sayings during EFT workshops is "The problem is never the problem." What I mean by this is that the problem we complain about today usually bothers us only because it resembles an earlier problem. For example, if your spouse being late disturbs you, you may discover by digging deep with EFT that the real reason this behavior triggers you is that your mother didn't meet your needs in early childhood. Your spouse's behavior in the present day resembles, to your brain, the neglect you experienced in early childhood, so you react accordingly. You put a lot of energy into trying to change your spouse when the present-day person is not the source of the problem.

On the EFT Universe website, we have published hundreds of stories in which someone was no longer triggered by a present problem after the emotional charge was removed from a similar childhood event. Nothing changed in the present day, yet the very problem that so vexed a person before now carries zero emotional charge. That's the magic that happens once we neutralize core issues with EFT. Rather than being content with using EFT on surface problems, it's worth developing the skills to find and resolve the core issues that are at the root of the problem.

Here are some questions you might ask in order to identify core issues:

- Does the problem that's bothering you remind you of any events in your childhood? Tune into your body and feel your feelings. Then travel back in time to the first time in your life you ever felt that same sensation.

- What's the worst similar experience you ever had?
- If you were writing your autobiography, what chapter would you prefer to delete, as though it had never happened to you?

If you can't remember a specific childhood event, simply make up a fictional event in your mind. This kind of guessing usually turns out to be right on target. You're assembling the imagined event out of components of real events, and the imaginary event usually leads back to actual events you can tap on. Even if it doesn't, and you tap on the fictional event, you will usually experience an obvious release of tension.

The Generalization Effect

The *generalization effect* is a phenomenon you'll notice as you make progress with EFT. As you resolve the emotional sting of specific events, other events with a similar emotional signature also decrease in intensity. I once worked with a man at an EFT workshop whose father had beaten him many times during his childhood. His SUD level on the beatings was a 10. I asked him to recall the worst beating he'd ever suffered. He told me that when he was eight years old, his father had hit him so hard he had broken the boy's jaw. We tapped together on that terrible beating, and after working on all the aspects, his SUD dropped to a 0. I asked him for a SUD score on all the beatings, and his face softened. He said, "My dad got beat by his dad much worse than he beat me. My dad actually did a pretty good job considering how badly he was raised." My client's SUD level on all the beatings dropped considerably after we reduced the intensity of this one beating. That's an example of EFT's generalization effect. When you knock down an important domino, all the other dominos can fall.

This is very reassuring to clients who suffered from many instances of childhood abuse, the way my client at that workshop had suffered. You don't need to work through every single horrible incident. Often, simply collapsing the emotional intensity behind one incident is sufficient to collapse the intensity around similar incidents.

The reason our brains work this way is because of a group of neurons in the emotional center of the brain, the limbic system, called the hippocampus. The hippocampus has the job of comparing one event to the other. Suppose that, as a five-year-old child in Catholic school, you get beaten by a nun. Forty years later, you can't figure out why you feel uneasy around women wearing outfits that are black and white. The reason for your adult aversion to a black-and-white combination is that the hippocampus associates the colors of the nun's habit with the pain of the beating.

This was a brilliant evolutionary innovation for your ancestors. Perhaps these early humans were attacked by a tiger hiding in the long grass. The tiger's stripes mimicked the patterns of the grass yet there was something different there. Learning to spot a pattern, judge the differences, and react with fear saved your alert ancestors.

They gave birth to their children, who also learned, just a little bit better, how to respond to threats. After thousands of generations, you have a hippocampus at the center of your brain that is genetically engineered to evaluate every message flooding in from your senses, and pick out those associated with the possibility of danger. You see the woman wearing the black-and-white cocktail dress at a party, your hippocampus associates these colors with the nun who beat you, and you have an emotional response.

Yet the opposite is also true. Assume for a moment you're a man who is very shy when confronted with women at cocktail parties. He feels a rush of fear whenever he thinks about talking to an attractive woman dressed in black. He works with an EFT coach on his memories of getting beaten by the nun in Catholic school, and suddenly he finds himself able to talk easily to women at parties. Once the man's hippocampus breaks the connection between beatings and a black dress, it knows, for future reference, that the two phenomena are no longer connected.

This is the explanation the latest brain science gives us for the generalization effect. It's been noted in EFT for many years, and it's very comforting for those who've suffered many adverse experiences. You may need to tap on some of them, but you won't have to tap on all of them before the whole group is neutralized. Sometimes, like my client who was beaten repeatedly as a child, if you tap on a big one, the generalization effect reduces the emotional intensity of all similar experiences.

The Movie Technique and Tell the Story Technique

When you take an EFT workshop, the first key technique you learn is the Movie Technique. Why do we place such emphasis on the Movie Technique? The reason for this is that it combines many of the methods that are key to success with EFT.

The first thing the Movie Technique does is focus you on being specific. EFT is great at eliminating the emotional intensity you feel, as long as it's used on an actual concrete event ("John yelled at me in the meeting"), rather than a general statement ("My procrastination").

The Movie Technique has you identify a particular incident that has a big emotional charge for you, and systematically reduce that charge to 0. You picture the event in your mind's eye just as though it were a movie, and run through the movie scene by scene.

Whenever you reach a part of the movie that carries a big emotional charge, you stop and perform the EFT sequence. In this way, you reduce the intensity of each of the bad parts of the movie. EFT's related technique, Tell the Story, is done out loud, while the Movie Technique is typically done silently. You can use the Movie Technique with a client without them ever disclosing what the event was.

Try this with one of your own traumatic life events right now. Think of the event as though it were a scary movie. Make sure it's an event that lasts just a few minutes; if your movie lasts several hours or days, you've probably picked a general pattern. Try again, selecting a different event, till you have a movie that's just a few minutes long.

One example is a man whose general issue is "Distrust of Strangers." We trace it to a particular childhood incident that occurred when the man, whom we'll call John, was seven years old. His parents moved to a new town, and John found himself walking to a new school through a rough neighborhood. He encountered a group of bullies at school but always managed to avoid them. One day, walking back from school, he saw the bullies walking toward him. He crossed the street, hoping to avoid their attention. He wasn't successful, and he saw them point at him, then change course to intercept him. He knew he was due for a beating. They taunted him and shoved him, and he fell into the gutter. His mouth hit the pavement, and he chipped a tooth. Other kids gathered round and laughed at him, and the bullies moved off. He picked himself up and walked the rest of the way home.

If you were to apply EFT to John's general pattern, "Distrust of Strangers," you'd be tapping generally—and ineffectually. When instead you focus on the specific event, you're honing in on the life events that gave rise to the general pattern. A collection of events like John's beating can combine to create the general pattern.

Now give your movie a title. John might call his movie "The Bullies."

Start thinking about the movie at a point before the traumatic part began. For John, that would be when he was walking home from school, unaware of the events in store for him.

Now run your movie through your mind till the end. The end of the movie is usually a place where the bad events come to an end. For John, this might be when he picked himself up off the ground, and resumed his walk home.

Now let's add EFT to your movie. Here's the way you do this:

1. Think of the title of your movie. Rate your degree of your emotional distress around just the title, not the movie itself. For instance, on the distress scale of 0 to 10 where 0 is no distress and 10 represents maximum distress, you might be an 8 when you think of the title "The Meeting." Write down your movie title, and your number.

2. Work the movie title into an EFT Setup Statement. It might sound something like this: "Even though [Insert Your Movie Title Here], I deeply and completely accept myself." Then tap on the EFT acupressure points, while repeating the Setup Statement three times. Your distress level will typically go down. You may have to do EFT several times on the title for it to reach a low number like 0 or 1 or 2.

3. Once the title reaches a low number, think of the "neutral point" before the bad events in the movie began to take place. For John, the neutral point was when he was walking home from school, before the bullies saw him. Once you've identified the neutral point of your own movie, start running the movie through your mind, until you reach a point where the emotional intensity rises. In John's case,

the first emotionally intense point was when he saw the bullies.

4. Stop at this point, and assess your intensity number. It might have risen from a 1 to a 7, for instance. Then perform a round of EFT on that first emotional crescendo. For John, it might be, "Even though I saw the bullies turn toward me, I deeply and completely accept myself." Use the same kind of statement for your own problem: "Even though [first emotional crescendo], I deeply and completely accept myself." Keep tapping till your number drops to 0 or near 0, perhaps a 1 or 2.

5. Now rewind your mental movie to the neutral point, and start running it in your mind again. Stop at the first emotional crescendo. If you sail right through the first one you tapped on, you know you've really and truly resolved that aspect of the memory with EFT. Go on to the next crescendo. For John, this might have been when they shoved him into the gutter. When you've found your second emotional crescendo, then repeat the process. Assess your intensity number, do EFT, and keep tapping till your number is low. Even if your number is only a 3 or 4, stop and do EFT again. Don't push through low-intensity emotional crescendos; since you have the gift of freedom at your fingertips, use it on each part of the movie.

6. Rewind to the neutral point again, and repeat the process.

7. When you can replay the whole movie in your mind, from the neutral point, to the end of the movie when

your feelings are neutral again, you'll know you've resolved the whole event. You'll have dealt with all the aspects of the traumatic incident.

8. To truly test yourself, run through the movie, but exaggerate each sensory channel. Imagine the sights, sounds, smells, tastes, and other aspects of the movie as vividly as you possible can. If you've been running the movie silently in your mind, speak it out loud. When you cannot possibly make yourself upset, you're sure to have resolved the lingering emotional impact of the event. The effect is usually permanent.

When you work through enough individual movies in this way, the whole general pattern often vanishes. Perhaps John had forty events that contributed to his distrust of strangers. He might need to do the Movie Technique on all forty, but experience with EFT suggests that when you resolve just a few key events, perhaps five or ten of them, the rest fade in intensity, and the general pattern itself is neutralized.

The Tell the Story Technique is similar to the Movie Technique; usually the Movie Technique is performed silently while Tell the Story is out loud. One great benefit of the Movie Technique done silently is that the client does not have to disclose the nature of the problem. An event might be too triggering, or too embarrassing, or too emotionally overwhelming, to be spoken out loud. That's no problem with the Movie Technique, which allows EFT to work its magic without the necessity of disclosure on the part of the client. The privacy offered by the Movie Technique makes it very useful for clients who would rather not talk openly about troubling events.

Constricted Breathing

Here's a way to demonstrate how EFT can affect you physically. You can try this yourself right now. It's also often practiced as an onstage demonstration at EFT workshops. You simply take three deep breaths, stretching your lungs as far as they can expand. On the third breath, rate the extent of the expansion of your lungs on a 0 to 10 scale, with 0 being as constricted as possible, and 10 being as expanded as possible. Now perform several rounds of EFT using Setup Statements such as:

Even though my breathing is constricted…

Even though my lungs will only expand to an 8…

Even though I have this physical problem that prevents me breathing deeply…

Now take another deep breath and rate your level of expansion. Usually there's substantial improvement. Now focus on any emotional contributors to constricted breathing. Use questions like:

What life events can I associate with breathing problems?

Are there places in my life where I feel restricted?

If I simply guess at an emotional reason for my constricted breathing, what might it be?

Now tap on any issues surfaced by these questions. After your intensity is reduced, take another deep breath and rate how far your lungs are now expanding. Even if you were a 10 earlier, you might now find you're an 11 or 14.

The Personal Peace Procedure

The Personal Peace Procedure consists of listing every specific troublesome event in your life and systematically using EFT to tap away the emotional impact of these events. With due diligence, you knock over every negative domino on your emotional playing board and, in so doing, remove significant sources of both emotional and physical ailments. You experience personal peace, which improves your work and home relationships, your health, and every other area of your life.

Tapping on large numbers of events one by one might seem like a daunting task, but we'll show you in the next few paragraphs how you can accomplish it quickly and efficiently. Because of EFT's generalization effect, where tapping on one issue reduces the intensity of similar issues, you'll typically find the process going much faster than you imagined.

Removing the emotional charge from your specific events results in less and less internal conflict. Less internal conflict results, in turn, in greater personal peace and less suffering on all levels—physical, mental, emotional, and spiritual. For many people, the Personal Peace Procedure has led to the complete cessation of lifelong

How to Do EFT: The Basic Recipe 71

issues that other methods did not resolve. You'll find stories on the EFT Universe website written by people who describe relief from physical maladies like headaches, breathing difficulties, and digestive disorders. You'll read other stories of people who used EFT to help them deal with the stress associated with AIDS, multiple sclerosis, and cancer. Unresolved anger, traumas, guilt, or grief contributes to physical illness, and cannot be medicated away. EFT addresses these emotional contributors to physical disease.

Here's how to do the Personal Peace Procedure:

1. List every specific troublesome event in your life that you can remember. Write them down in a Personal Peace Procedure journal. "Troublesome" means it caused you some form of discomfort. If you listed fewer than fifty events, try harder to remember more. Many people find hundreds. Some bad events you recall may not seem to cause you any current discomfort. List them anyway. The fact that they came to mind suggests they may need resolution. As you list them, give each specific event a title, like it's a short movie, such as: Mom slapped me that time in the car; I stole my brother's baseball cap; I slipped and fell in front of everybody at the ice skating rink; My third grade class ridiculed me when I gave that speech; Dad locked me in the toolshed overnight; Mrs. Simmons told me I was dumb.

2. When your list is finished, choose the biggest dominoes on your board, that is, the events that have the most emotional charge for you. Apply EFT to them,

one at a time, until the SUD level for each event is 0. You might find yourself laughing about an event that used to bring you to tears; you might find a memory fading. Pay attention to any aspects that arise and treat them as separate dominoes, by tapping for each aspect separately. Make sure you tap on each event until it is resolved. If you find yourself unable to rate the intensity of a bad event on the 0-10 scale, you might be dissociating, or repressing a memory. One solution to this problem is to tap ten rounds of EFT on every aspect of the event you are able to recall. You might then find the event emerging into clearer focus but without the same high degree of emotional charge.

3. After you have removed the biggest dominoes, pick the next biggest, and work on down the line.

4. If you can, clear at least one of your specific events, preferably three, daily for three months. By taking only minutes per day, in three months you will have cleared 90 to 270 specific events. You will likely discover that your body feels better, that your threshold for getting upset is much lower, your relationships have improved, and many of your old issues have disappeared. If you revisit specific events you wrote down in your Personal Peace Procedure journal, you will likely discover that the former intensity has evaporated. Pay attention to improvements in your blood pressure, pulse, and respiratory capacity. EFT often produces subtle but measurable changes

in your health, and you may miss them if you aren't looking for them.

5. After knocking down all your dominoes, you may feel so much better that you're tempted to alter the dosages of medications your doctor has prescribed. Never make any such changes without consulting with your physician. Your doctor is your partner in your healing journey. Tell your doctor that you're working on your emotional issues with EFT, since most health-care professionals are acutely aware of the contribution that stress makes to disease.

The Personal Peace Procedure does not take the place of EFT training, nor does it take the place of assistance from a qualified EFT practitioner. It is an excellent supplement to EFT workshops and help from EFT practitioners. EFT's full range of resources is designed to work effectively together for the best healing results.

Is It Working Yet?

Sometimes EFT's benefits are blindingly obvious. In the introductory video on the home page of the EFT Universe website, you see a TV reporter with a lifelong fear of spiders receiving a tapping session. Afterward, in a dramatic turnaround, she's able to stroke a giant hairy tarantula spider she's holding in the palm of her hand.

Other times, EFTs effects are subtler and you have to pay close attention to spot them. A friend of mine who has had a lifelong fear of driving in high-speed traffic remarked to me recently that her old fear is completely gone. Over the past year, each time she felt anxious about driving, she pulled her car to the side of the road and tapped. It took many trips and much tapping, but subtle changes gradually took effect. Thanks to EFT she has emotional freedom and drives without fear. She also has another great benefit, in the form of a closer bond to her daughter and baby granddaughter. They live two hours drive away and, previously, her dread of traffic kept her from visiting them. Now she's able to make the drive with joyful anticipation of playing with her granddaughter.

If you seem not to be making progress on a particular problem despite using EFT, look for other positive changes that might be happening in your life. Stress affects every system in the body, and once you relieve it with EFT, you might find improvements in unexpected areas. For instance, when stressed, the capillaries in your digestive system constrict, impeding digestion. Many people with digestive problems report improvement after EFT. Stress also redistributes biological resources away from your reproductive system. You'll find many stories on EFT Universe of people whose sex lives improved dramatically as a by-product of healing emotional issues. Stress affects your muscular and circulatory systems; many people report that muscular aches and pains disappear after EFT, and their blood circulation improves. Just as stress is pervasive, relaxation is pervasive, and when we release our emotional bonds with EFT, the relaxing effects are felt all over the body. So perhaps your sore knee has only improved slightly, but you're sleeping better, having fewer respiratory problems, and getting along better with your coworkers.

Saying the Right Words

A common misconception is that you have to say just the right words while tapping in order for EFT to be effective. The truth is that focusing on the problem is more important than the exact words you're using. It's the exposure to the troubling issue that directs healing energy to the right place; the words are just a guide.

Many practitioners write down tapping scripts with lists of affirmations you can use. These can be useful. However, your own words are usually able to capture the full intensity of your emotions in a way that is not possible using other people's words. The way you form language is associated with the configuration of the neural network in your brain. You want the neural pathways along which stress signals travel to be very active while you tap. Using your own words is more likely to awaken that neural pathway fully than using even the most eloquent words suggested by someone else. By all means use tapping scripts if they're available, to nudge you in the right direction. At the same time, utilize the power of prolonged exposure by focusing your mind completely on your own experience. Your mind and body have a healing wisdom that usually directs healing power toward the place where it is most urgently required.

The Next Steps on Your EFT Journey

Now that you've entered the world of EFT, you'll find it to be a rich and supportive place. On the EFT Universe website, you'll find stories written by thousands of people, from all over the world, describing success with an enormous variety of problems. Locate success stories on your particular problem by using the site's drop-down menu, which lists issues alphabetically: Addictions, ADHD, Anxiety, Depression, and so on. Read these stories for insights on how to apply EFT to your particular case. They'll inspire you in your quest for full healing.

Our certified practitioners are a wonderful resource. They've gone through rigorous training in Clinical EFT and have honed their skills with many clients. Many of them work via telephone or videoconferencing, so if you don't find the perfect practitioner in your geographic area, you can still get expert help with remote sessions. While EFT is primarily a self-help tool and you can get great results alone, you'll find the insight that comes from an outside observer can often alert you to behavior patterns and solutions you can't find by yourself.

Take an EFT workshop. EFT Universe offers more than a hundred workshops each year, all over the world, and you're likely to find a Level 1 and 2 workshop close to you. You'll make friends, see expert demonstrations, and learn EFT systematically. Each workshop contains eight learning modules, and each module builds on the one before. Fifteen years' experience in training thousands of people in EFT has shown us exactly how people learn EFT competently and quickly, and provided the background knowledge to design these trainings. Read the many testimonials on the website to see how deeply transformational the EFT workshops are.

The EFT Universe newsletter is the medium that keeps the whole EFT world connected. Read the stories

How to Do EFT: The Basic Recipe

published there weekly to stay inspired and to learn about new uses for EFT. Write your own experiences and submit them to the newsletter. Post comments on the EFT Universe Facebook page, and comment in the blogs.

If you'd like to help others access the benefits you have gained from EFT, you might consider volunteering your services. There are dozens of ways to support EFT's growth and progress. You can join a tapping circle, or start one yourself. You can donate to EFT research and humanitarian efforts. You can offer tapping sessions to people who are suffering through one of EFT's humanitarian projects, like those that have reached thousands in Haiti, Rwanda, and elsewhere. You can let your friends know about EFT.

EFT has reached millions of people worldwide with its healing magic but is still in its infancy. By reading this book and practicing this work, you're joining a healing revolution that has the potential to radically reduce human suffering. Imagine if the benefits you've already experienced could be shared by every child, every sick person, every anxious or stressed person in the world. The trajectory of human history would be very different. I'm committed to helping create this shift however I can, and I invite you to join me and all the other people of goodwill in making this vision of a transformed future a reality.

3

Tapping Options and Variations

In many, if not most cases, the Basic Recipe is all you need for successful resolution of the issues for which you are using EFT. In some cases, for example, when a SUD level refuses to budge from a plateau of 2 while using the "shortcut" (the Basic Recipe), returning to EFT's original formula, called the Full Basic Recipe, may bring it down to the desired 0. Some clients and practitioners simply prefer to use the Full Basic Recipe as a matter of course. Once you learn it, you'll find that it doesn't take that much longer than the shorter Basic Recipe.

The Full Basic Recipe includes a curious technique called the 9 Gamut Procedure. In this chapter, you will learn that procedure, the sequence of the full recipe, and additional optional points that you might find helpful in your tapping.

Here are the parts that make up the Full Basic Recipe:

1. The Setup Statement (tap on the Karate Chop point or rub the Sore Spot).

2. The tapping sequence (tap on the sequence of 7 or 12 points).
3. The 9 Gamut Procedure.
4. The tapping sequence again.

Alternative to the Karate Chop Point: The Sore Spot

In chapter 2, you learned to tap on the Karate Chop point while saying the Setup Statement ("Even though I have ____, I deeply and completely accept myself"). As an alternative, you can instead rub what is called "the Sore Spot." This spot is located on your upper chest and, like all the EFT points, there is one on each side of your body (see illustration). You can rub on either of the two. The spot gets its name from the fact that this place is tender to the touch

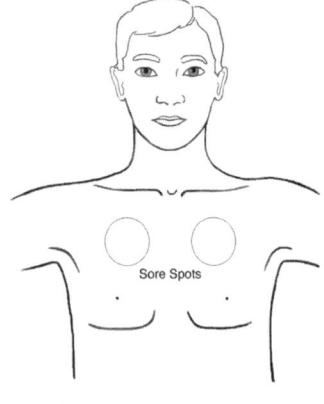

The Sore Spot

The Sore Spot is located two or three inches below the notch at the base of your throat (just above your sternum) and to the left or right on your chest two or three inches. If you probe with your fingers in that region, you will feel a place where there is some tenderness. This Sore Spot is where you rub while saying the Setup Statement, just as you did while tapping on the Karate Chop point. It's up to you which one you use. Using either the Sore Spot or the Karate Chop point is correct, just as using either one of the Sore Spots is fine. You may have had chest surgery, so can only rub on one of the Sore Spots, or use only the Karate Chop point. That is fine too. As always, if you have a medical condition and are uncertain about the advisability of the physical aspects of tapping, consult your health-care provider.

The Tapping Sequence for the Full Basic Recipe

After saying the Setup Statement three times, either tapping on the Karate Chop point or rubbing the Sore Spot, here is the tapping sequence you will use for the Full Basic Recipe. You start with the same seven points you learned in the Basic Recipe, add five more points, and end by tapping on the Karate Chop point.

1. Beginning of the Eyebrow (EB)
2. Side of the Eye (SE)
3. Under the Eye (UE)
4. Under the Nose (UN)
5. Chin (Ch)
6. Beginning of the Collarbone (CB)
7. Under the Arm (UA)

Add these five points in this order:

8. Below the Nipple (BN)
9. Thumb (Th)
10. Index Finger (IF)
11. Middle Finger (MF)
12. Baby Finger (BF)

Karate Chop (KC)

The following are illustrations of the five new points. As with the other points, there is one on each side of the body. Either side is fine to use. In the case of the Below the Nipple point, some people tap on both at once. In the case of the hand points, you can use one side, alternate sides, or use the point on one hand to tap on the same point on the other hand. It's up to you which way you choose to do it. Go with what feels most comfortable. That will increase the likelihood of your continuing to use EFT and achieving the relief you seek from problems that have been plaguing you.

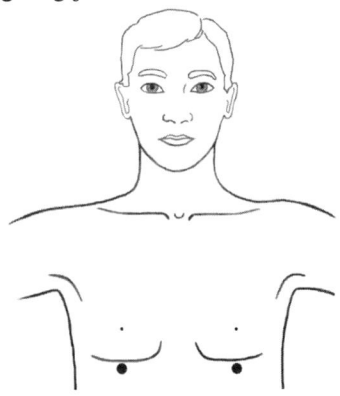

Below the Nipple (BN) Points

Tapping Options and Variations   83

Below the Nipple: For men, this point is an inch below the nipple. For women, this point is below the nipple where the elastic of a bra runs beneath the breasts.

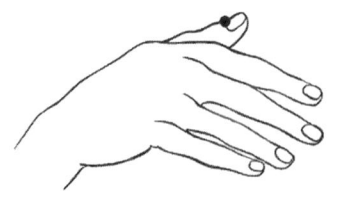

Thumb (Th) Point

Thumb: This point is on the side of the thumb away from the hand at the level of the base of the thumbnail.

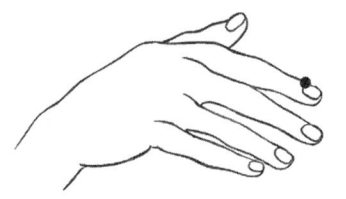

Index Finger (IF) Point

Index Finger: This point is on the side of the index finger nearest the thumb at the level of the base of the fingernail.

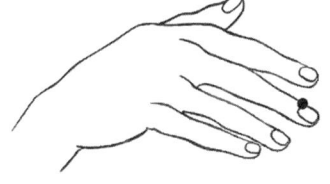

Middle Finger (MF) Point

Middle Finger: This point is on the side of the middle finger nearest the index finger at the level of the base of the fingernail.

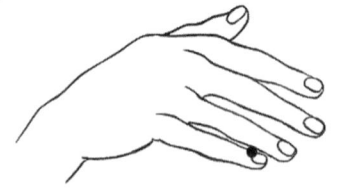

Baby Finger (BF) Point

Baby Finger: This point is on the side of the baby finger nearest the middle finger at the level of the base of the fingernail.

Note that one finger is omitted in the hand tapping points. It is not necessary to include the ring finger, but some EFTers tap on the same place on that finger as on the other fingers because it is simply easier to include all. That's fine too. It won't hurt anything to add some extra tapping!

After the Setup Statement and the first round of tapping, the Full Basic Recipe proceeds to the 9 Gamut Procedure.

The 9 Gamut Procedure and Eye Movements

One of the oddest-looking parts of EFT is the 9 Gamut Procedure. It involves tapping on a point on the back of the hand, the Gamut point (see illustration), while moving your eyes in a circle, as well as to the side. Though the technique appears odd, research has demonstrated that eye movements are key to reprocessing old traumatic memories.

The University of South Florida conducted a study of people with posttraumatic stress disorder (PTSD) and depression, using a new method called Accelerated Resolution Therapy (ART). They found that ART rapidly reduced the emotional charge held in memories of traumatic events. ART uses eye movements, and also has clients visualize a desired outcome. Participants in the study experienced dramatic drops in both PTSD and depression symptoms, as well as improved sleep. The study was published in the journal *Behavioral Sciences*.

Another study, published in the journal *Traumatology*, was a collaboration between a psychiatrist and an optician. They were colleagues who happened upon the discovery that when traumatized people remember an emotionally charged event, they are unable to maintain stable peripheral vision; their eyes flutter when turned hard right or left. After successful psychiatric treatment and the traumatized individuals are able to recall the event without emotional distress, the fluttering disappears.

Neuroscientists don't know exactly why this association between traumatic memories and eye movements occurs. It may be linked to the ability of the brain to process a disturbing event. The midbrain or limbic system contains structures that are responsible for turning short-term memories into long-term ones. This memory-processing function is impaired in patients suffering from PTSD.

Experience with tens of thousands of clients has shown the 9 Gamut Procedure to be effective even when the other parts of EFT's Basic Recipe are unable to provide resolution to a problem. During Clinical EFT training and certification, the 9 Gamut Procedure is emphasized; slow eye movements covering every point in the field of peripheral vision are found to be particularly valuable. The 9 Gamut Procedure often helps with:

- Disturbing emotions that can't be linked to a specific event.
- Traumatic incidents that occurred very early in a person's life, before memory formation began (usually around age 4).
- When there are a great many similar traumatic events, such as frequent childhood beatings.
- Womb trauma. Stress hormones such as cortisol and adrenaline cross the placental barrier; a child may be "learning" stress at the level of molecular conditioning even before birth.
- Clients whose SUD level is not going down using EFT's shortcut Basic Recipe.

For all these reasons, backed by the emerging science linking eye movements to memory reconsolidation, the 9 Gamut Procedure is useful for anyone using EFT to know and it is an essential part of every EFT practitioner's toolkit.

The 9 Gamut Procedure is so named because you perform nine simple actions while tapping on the Gamut point.

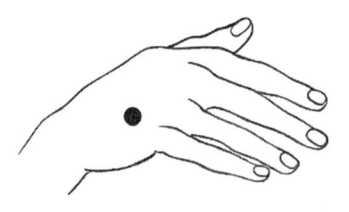

The Gamut Point

The Gamut point is on the back of either hand in the shallow between the ligaments extending from the ring finger and the little finger, about a half-inch toward the wrist from the knuckles. If you tap in that area with the three fingers of your other hand, you are bound to hit the point!

While tapping on the Gamut point, here are the nine actions you perform in order:

1. Close your eyes.
2. Open your eyes.
3. Look down hard right (without moving your head).
4. Look down hard left (without moving your head).
5. Roll your eyes in a full clockwise circle, again without moving your head.
6. Roll your eyes in a full counterclockwise circle, without moving your head.
7. Hum two seconds of a song (such as "Row, Row, Row Your Boat" or "Happy Birthday").
8. Count rapidly from 1 to 5.
9. Hum two seconds of a song again.

It may seem like a lot to remember at first, but after you've done it a few times, you will find that you can accomplish the nine actions quickly and easily. Though the actions may seem arbitrary, there is a purpose to each. As explained previously, there is a link between eye movements and the neural pathways of traumatic memories. As for humming a song, it activates the right brain (the creative side of the brain), while counting activates the left brain (the logical, reasoning side).

Some EFT practitioners have discovered that using "Happy Birthday" as the song to hum can raise unhappy birthday memories in clients, thus interfering with the EFT work at hand. For this reason, some use "Row, Row, Row Your Boat" instead. Again, it's up to you what you decide to hum. Make it something easy and automatic, however. Thinking about what to hum takes you out of your right brain into your left, and defeats the purpose!

Some Optional Points

Since the development of EFT, many variations have emerged, including the addition of acupuncture points that are not part of the traditional Full Basic Recipe. As mentioned, it doesn't hurt to add more points to the tapping sequence. Many EFTers and practitioners regularly include the following points. It is not necessary for you to use them, but you may have fun trying them out. If you decide to add them to your standard tapping sequence, it is a good idea to get comfortable with the basic seven or twelve points first. Overwhelming yourself with points to remember might deter you from integrating EFT into your daily life and discovering the full benefits of this simple technique.

Top of the Head: This is the highest point on your head, which is not the exact center of the top of your head, but slightly back from the center.

Wrists: There are acupuncture meridians running through the inside and outside of your wrists. When you tap on the fingers and thumb in the Full Basic Recipe, you are tapping on endpoints of these meridians. Some practitioners have their clients slap gently on the inside (at the base of the palm) and then the outside (at the base of the back of the hand) of either wrist instead of tapping on the thumb and finger points. This addresses all the thumb and finger meridians at once. Again, either way is fine: tap on your hand points or gently slap both sides of your wrist. You can also cover all of the wrist points at once by tapping one wrist against the other, first with the insides together then with the outsides together.

Ankles: As with the wrists, meridians run through the ankles. Though perhaps not as convenient to tap on as the wrists, the ankle points are part of many EFTers' tapping protocol. To address these points, tap on the front and back of either or both ankles. As with the wrists, you can also cross your ankles and tap one against the other, front to back, then switch to cross and tap with the other foot in front.

The Tendency to Explain Away EFT's Positive Effects

A phenomenon that often occurs in the use of EFT is the tendency not to acknowledge the effectiveness of EFT either through coming up with various explanations for why it worked (a common one is "The tapping distracted me from my problem") or denial that the problem was that bad to begin with. This tendency to explain away the positive results is known as the "apex effect" or "apex problem," as clinical psychologist Dr. Roger Callahan termed it.

It can be difficult for people to accept that this simple method of tapping could have resolved their physical, emotional, or behavioral problem, especially if they'd had the problem for years. Faced with the quick or relatively quick resolution of the problem, the mind cannot grasp how this could possibly be. After trying a dozen other methods, after ten years of psychotherapy, after taking every medication imaginable—how could my problem have gone away? The mind, not understanding how EFT works, casts around for logical explanations in its own realm of experience, which before this has not included energy medicine. With nothing to compare the experience to, the mind comes up with a range of reasons, none of which are all that logical.

Denying that the problem wasn't that serious is one way to explain the "illogical" results of the tapping. The denial may not be purposeful. Sometimes the person really doesn't remember that it was a serious problem before applying EFT to it. This is actually a common occurrence with EFT. The emotional upset associated with an event disappears so effectively that the person can hardly remember what was so upsetting about the event. This is one of the reasons we use the SUD scale. Writing down the intensity of your feeling before you start tapping gives you concrete evidence of the severity of your problem. Writing down your ending SUD level shows how effective the tapping really was. Keeping a tapping journal is a good idea. That way, if you find yourself minimizing the severity of the problem you tapped for, you can pull out the journal to remind yourself of just how well this simple technique is working.

To help your mind integrate the effectiveness of energy medicine, you might want to go to the research pages on the EFT Universe website. There you can satisfy your mind's quest for a logical explanation for this "strange" thing called tapping.

The reason for this discussion is to prepare you for the apex effect so you don't let it stop you from continuing to use EFT. Even if you're thinking EFT makes no sense, consult the numbers in your tapping journal to remind you how much it is helping, and keep tapping. You don't have to believe in it for it to be effective. That's a wonderful feature of EFT!

Another great feature is that you don't have to do it perfectly for it to work. If you forget a point or tap the points out of order, you will likely still get results. So don't worry about getting it just right. Keep reviewing the points and keep tapping. With use, the tapping points and the sequences to follow for the Basic Recipe and the Full Basic Recipe will become second nature to you.

Practicing the Full Basic Recipe

Now that you have learned the parts of the Full Basic Recipe, let's review it using a sample problem. To keep it simple, we'll stick to a physical symptom—shoulder pain. You can use this same basic script, however, to address other aspects of fibromyalgia and chronic fatigue, including depression and anxiety.

- State the problem: I have pain in both my shoulder joints.
- How bad is it? It's really painful. On a scale from 1 to 10, the pain is an 8.
- Setup: Tap on the Karate Chop point or rub the Sore Spot while saying:

  Even though I have this shoulder pain, I fully and completely accept myself.

  Even though I have this shoulder pain, I fully and completely accept myself.

  Even though I have this shoulder pain, I fully and completely accept myself.

- The Sequence: Tap on the twelve points of the Full Basic Recipe while repeating your Reminder Phrase: *This shoulder pain.* End by saying the Reminder Phrase while tapping on the Karate Chop point.
- 9 Gamut Procedure: Tap on the Gamut point while doing the following:
  1. Close your eyes.
  2. Open your eyes.
  3. Look down hard right (without moving your head).
  4. Look down hard left (without moving your head).

Tapping Options and Variations

5. Roll your eyes in a full clockwise circle, again without moving your head.
6. Roll your eyes in a full counterclockwise circle, without moving your head.
7. Hum two seconds of a song (such as "Row, Row, Row Your Boat" or "Happy Birthday").
8. Count rapidly from 1 to 5.
9. Hum two seconds of a song again.

- Repeat the Sequence: Tap on the twelve points and the KC point while saying your Reminder Phrase.

That's it—the Full Basic Recipe. Now measure your progress on the 0-10 scale. How does your shoulder pain feel now? If it is completely gone, down to 0, you need do no more on this symptom. For illustration's sake, let's say your pain has dropped from an 8 to a 3. Your shoulders feel somewhat better, but the pain is still there. Do another round of the Full Basic Recipe, using slightly modified language.

- Adjusted Setup: Tap on the Karate Chop point or rub the Sore Spot while saying:

    Even though I still have some shoulder pain, I fully and completely accept myself.

    Even though I still have some shoulder pain, I fully and completely accept myself.

    Even though I still have some shoulder pain, I fully and completely accept myself.

- The Sequence: Tap on the twelve points and the Karate Chop point while saying your modified Reminder Phrase: This remaining shoulder pain.
- 9 Gamut Procedure: Tap the Gamut point while doing the following:
- Repeat the Sequence: Tap on the twelve points and the KC point while saying your modified Reminder Phrase: This remaining shoulder pain.
- Rate your pain on the SUD scale again. If you are still not at a 0, tap through the Full Basic Recipe again.

Tapping directly on physical pain, as we did in the example here, is the easiest way to learn EFT. It is important to note, however, that EFT is most effective when you address the emotional components of your physical pain, or any other problem. You may be able to tap your pain down to the lower numbers on the SUD scale simply by doing tapping rounds on the pain, but getting your number to 0 may require using EFT to uncover and clear the emotional aspects of your pain. The basics are the same.

You now have the tools you need to use EFT to address any symptom or aspect of your fibromyalgia, chronic fatigue, Lyme disease, or other autoimmune conditions.

4

Tapping for Fibromyalgia as a Spiritual Energy Imbalance

by Rue Anne Hass, MA, EFT Founding Master

There is often a deeper truth underlying fibromyalgia and chronic fatigue, which makes successful treatment of these conditions using conventional medicine difficult or even unlikely. The process of EFT can help you uncover that truth.

In the realm of traditional Chinese medicine, the medical system in which acupuncture is a primary technique, fibromyalgia could be called a "disharmony of the spirit." Think about this phrase as you read the following descriptions of two "typical" fibromyalgia sufferers:*

> Eight years ago, Tammy worked as an office manager and had three young children. Then her husband died, and her children began to have problems adjusting at school. A single working mother with a stressful job, Tammy would lie awake at night worrying about her situation. "My sleep went off first," she recalled. "I'd never had trouble falling asleep before,

---

*Examples adapted from www.tcmpage.com/hpfibromyalgia.html.

but I would lie awake night after night, thinking about my kids and my job, and it seemed that I never had a deep, sound sleep, even if I dozed off. After a while I would wake up in the morning feeling stiff all over and extremely tired. When I went to see my doctor he gave me an antidepressant, but it didn't work, plus I gained weight." Gradually, Tammy's condition worsened.

Sheila is an elementary school teacher. Six years ago, her twenty-four-year marriage ended in a bitter divorce. Four years ago, she was diagnosed with fibromyalgia. She had multiple complaints: fatigue, depression, muscle aches, insomnia, irritable bowel syndrome, and poor memory. She always woke up between 1:00 a.m. and 3:00 a.m., feeling restless and remembering a lot of dreams. She has always driven herself to excel in her work, but, these days, she is finding it very stressful and often thinks that she can't handle it anymore.

Both Tammy and Sheila were in pain and having trouble sleeping. Tammy was mostly worried, whereas Sheila's emotional tone contained more anger. Both had responded to the life conditions that befell them by tightening up inside. Acupuncturists say, "Wherever there is pain, there is no free flow of energy. Where there is no pain, there is free flow of energy." Perhaps Tammy and Sheila's inner tightness, which interferes with energy flow, led to the development of their fibromyalgia symptoms.

At the deepest level, however, I believe that both Tammy and Sheila were experiencing a disharmony of spirit, a constriction of their self-expression, the natural free flow of energy in the body, mind, and spirit.

Three Different Perspectives on Fibromyalgia

Conventional Medical Perspective

- Fibromyalgia is a syndrome diagnosis (many different recurring symptoms under one name).
- Fibromyalgia is a complex nervous system pain disorder (shows up in many ways in the nervous system).
- Abnormal brain activity starts with a trigger but does not return to normal when the trigger is no longer present. The trigger may be repeated over time. This brain response may be adaptive for protection.
- The sensitive temperament is able to regulate physical and emotional responses only when there is very low stimulation in the person's environment.

Psychospiritual Perspective

- Chronic emotional and physical pain is obstructed spiritual energy, a constriction of the heart, reflected as pain in the body.
- Some of the essential qualities of spirit are love, expansiveness, generosity, creativity, imagination, possibility, openness, growth, flow, and purpose.
- A sensitive person may feel unable to fully express his or her true self in what feels like a harsh, critical, wounding world.
- As a result of life traumas, a sensitive person may eventually respond by constricting his or her whole

being around a thought: "I can't express what I really feel, I can't be who I really am, I am not good enough. In order to matter or have significance, in order to have inner peace, and in order to justify taking care of myself, I must be ill."

Energy Psychology Perspective

- In EFT and other energy methods, we are working with the energy meridian system as described by traditional Chinese medicine (TCM).

- Fibromyalgia is a Western diagnosis that has been used to label a condition that can manifest in TCM as several different patterns of imbalance. When we approach a problem energetically, we are engaging with a specific pattern that is manifesting in the body, without trying to label it as a diagnosis.

- Emotions like sadness and anger constrict the flow of energy (*qi* or *chi*) in our bodies, which can cause blockages and imbalance in body and organ systems. Lack of free flow can present as pain. The body can become ill.

- Fibromyalgia could be called an interruption in a particularly sensitive person's electrical system resulting from emotional trauma.

- Repeated experiences of stress or trauma can disrupt the energy system and restrict the flow of life, limiting access to our capacity to think and act and make choices.

- If, over time, we repress the emotions (sadness, anger, fear) that arise in response to our traumatic experi-

Fibromyalgia as a Spiritual Energy Imbalance

ences, the disruption in the electrical system is likely to show up as pain and dis-ease in the body.

- In TCM, the Heart is called the master of the organs. The Heart houses the Spirit. Clearing the disruption with energy techniques can clear the pain, change thought, change behavior, and open the Heart, resulting in healing.

These three ways of describing fibromyalgia are different ways of describing an *obstruction or a tightening* — the "not-free-flow" — that is happening throughout the body-mind-spirit system.

The "pain of the spirit" means to me that the person is restricting the free flow of his or her life expression. In the case of the earlier examples, Tammy is constricting around *worry and fear,* and Sheila is constricting around anger.

Pain in the physical body can be a signal that we have been holding worry, fear, and anger inside for a long time.

Fibromyalgia as a Disharmony of Spirit

My colleague Dr. Nancy Selfridge, with whom I taught classes on fibromyalgia, has said, "Doctors don't know what to do with their fibro patients. Physicians hate to be unsuccessful, and they are almost always unsuccessful when they try to heal fibromyalgia with conventional medicine."

While fibromyalgia is puzzling to medical science, it makes perfect spiritual sense.

There is a quality of energy or presence that each of us carries with us throughout our days. That energy, as it expresses through us in ways unique to each of us, has the capacity to form empowering, nourishing, cocreative, and liberating connections.

I believe that, as humans, we are open flowing systems, capable of drawing in and transforming energy from the infinite into the particular. Our actions and our choices form our individual bodies and lives. We are also able to flow our own energy from ourselves into the infinite.

Often, however, we hold within ourselves smaller "systems" of energy that are more closed than open. This diminishes the open flow of our energy. The overall effect is that we feel isolated, separated, and alienated from the cosmos around us.

When we have a wound, a memory, a rigid habit, a restrictive belief, it is as if we constrict ourselves around it. Like the grain of sand in an oyster, these "particles" of ourselves are where we become less flowing, less open, more self-protective, or even self-denying. In the very act of living each day, we run into situations that can cause such constrictions.

But suppose we are constricted around being ourselves? Suppose we view the very idea of being a self, of being a unique person—of being a person at all—as a condition of separation and constriction? Suppose I feel shame, for instance, about being a human being, or about deserving to take up space in the world. Or suppose that

Fibromyalgia as a Spiritual Energy Imbalance

I struggle with having a physical body with its passions, appetites, instincts, fleshiness, and so on. Then I cease to be as open a system as I might be. The flow of life energy, of light, of power within me is diminished. At that point, all the other ways I create constriction and obstructions in my life become that much more powerful, that much more difficult to work with.

In the same way, when for some reason we feel alienated from ourselves, or that our "self" is a condition of, or a reason for, constriction, it is like a metaphysical attack of asthma. If this feeling is denied or "stuffed" so we don't have to feel it, it can show up in the body as pain.

Even though it is not yet scientifically possible to prove this, there is ample clinical evidence that the symptoms of any disease in the body can be framed as a response to some form of inner mental, emotional, and spiritual constriction. Fibromyalgia is a perfect example of a "spiritual dis-ease" in the body-mind-spirit system. The symptoms of fibromyalgia are fatigue, sleep disruption, pain, and depression. As Gary Craig said to me once, "Fibromyalgia is to the body like low self-esteem is to the personality."

Much of our religious heritage implies that the soul is "somewhere else," resident in a different realm from the body. I believe that the body is an aspect of the soul, that the body is "distilled soul," as it were. Wouldn't it make sense that the fatigue, pain, and sadness of fibromyalgia are physical and emotional responses to, or maybe a mirror of, our blocked joy, love, and creative spiritual expression?

An original meaning of the word "breath," in ancient languages such as Aramaic and Hebrew, is "spirit." You could say that the movement of spirit and life throughout the cosmos is the "breath of God," the respiration of cocreation. Ideally, this breath should move in us and through us freely. We are each a "lung of the sacred," and we expand and contract so that spirit moves freely and empoweringly through us to all the world.

We can learn to reimagine ourselves, see ourselves as sacred, spiritual beings, not in spite of but because of being here. To incarnate is a divine activity. After all, the cosmos is an incarnation, the original one, and all other incarnations, manifestations, and expressions of life replicate it.

We can learn to experience ourselves in a way that expands us, and restores us to a feeling of openness and flow. It doesn't mean we become completely free of wounds, challenges, problems, pains, doubts, and all the rest of those feelings and experiences that constrict us. It does mean that these constrictions take place within a larger context of flow. They are capable of being healed, transformed, and restored to openness and flow themselves.

Then we can engage and cocreate with others in ways that feel right to us. Then our actions and choices can carry and assist the power of the flowing energy of the universe itself. This is true healing.

I believe that fibromyalgia is a message to our humanity—indeed, a cry to the best in us, to say that we are selling ourselves short. People with fibromyalgia are like the canary in the coal mine. Remember how the old-time miners used to send a canary in a cage down into the mine to see if there was enough oxygen down there to support life? If the canary lived, the miners would be sent down to work. If the canary died, well, I guess it was too bad for the canary...

Perhaps, like all illness, fibromyalgia in our times is a message that our bodies are sending to our conscious awareness: "We are not getting enough spirit in here! Open up! Relax and enjoy yourself! Live your purpose."

How to Tap for a Disharmony of Spirit

As tappers, our underlying premise is that the flow and balance of the body's electromagnetic, subtle energies are important for physical, spiritual, and emotional health, and for fostering well-being. EFT works within the ancient Chinese meridian system to balance the whole energy system.

If we start tapping for fibromyalgia by saying the Setup Phrase, "Even though I have fibromyalgia, I deeply and completely accept myself," all kinds of inner objections may instantly pop into our minds. We may find ourselves thinking, "How can I accept myself? I have so many flaws. I am just not good enough. I hate this pain. I am so angry with my body for doing this to me! Why can't I just get rid of this? What is wrong with me? This illness must be a punishment."

The Setup Phrase might be a starting point, but it is really only useful at the beginning to uncover all the beliefs and feelings that lie under it. How we feel about having fibromyalgia is a big clue to how we feel about ourselves. Harboring those feelings may be contributing to the syndrome of fibromyalgia.

Tapping for fibromyalgia means reaching to the deepest levels of how we think about ourselves and what is possible for us in the world. When we tap, we are not "treating" fibromyalgia in the Western medical sense or as a TCM doctor would. We are tapping for the specific pattern of energetic constriction in our bioelectric field that is showing up as our physical discomfort, our feelings, our beliefs, and our self-talk. Each person with fibromyalgia is unique.

A good place to start is to tap for the pain.

After you tap for the pain itself, try asking yourself: "If this pain, or discomfort, or these tears had a voice, what would this voice be saying?" This question will bring up many feelings, thoughts, images, and beliefs that you can incorporate into your tapping.

When we really listen to what our symptoms are saying, they want us to change our lives, and change how we think about and talk about ourselves. Inner balance and harmony will follow our thoughts. Tapping can open the door for harmony at all of our energetic levels. But it requires that we allow our lives to change deeply, too. For many people, that is the hard part.

Meridian System Imbalances

You probably know already that each energy meridian or pathway is part of a network and each is related to a body organ or, more accurately, a function. Unlike Western medicine, TCM considers the functions in our body, rather than specific organs. Each function embodies a way of thinking, a story about what is happening inside us, physically, mentally, emotionally, and spiritually. This story reflects and tells about our way of responding to life.

For example, insomnia is common among people who suffer from fibromyalgia and related syndromes. In TCM, insomnia is a message about an inner energetic imbalance of the fundamental substances (called by acupuncturists chi, blood, yin, yang, jing, and shen) or of the major organ systems (Lung, Heart, Spleen, Liver, and Kidney).

Many TCM practitioners believe that when a person suffers from insomnia, the two organ systems that are most often out of balance are the Heart and the Liver. (Note that when I capitalize these terms, I am referring to the meridian of that name rather than just the organ that the meridian regulates.) Each of these organ systems houses an aspect of the spirit. If the function of these organ systems is in disharmony, they may not be able to house the spirit properly, and the spirit may "wander."

The Energetic Pattern of the Spleen

Many people who suffer with fibromyalgia have digestive disturbances, and a life-long pattern of worrying and "swallowing their feelings." In the energy terms of TCM, a key to fibromyalgia is the Spleen meridian. One of the Spleen meridian's functions is to partner with the Stomach meridian on the way to nourishing the Heart. The Spleen, according to TCM, also nourishes muscles, which explains the occurrence of muscle pain in fibromyalgia.

Western medical facts are consistent with the TCM view. The spleen organ "recycles" the blood; that is, it filters the blood, removing old or damaged red blood cells and bacterial or viral pathogens to protect against infection. The spleen also functions as reserve storage for blood. Since red blood cells transport oxygen, which is what every cell needs to make its own energy to function, the spleen really does hold the nourishment for the heart and the muscle tissue!

In their article "Chinese Medicine for Fibromyalgia" (see www.tcmpage.com/hpfibromyalgia.html), Wei Liu, TCMD, MPH, LAc, and Changzhen Gong, PhD, MS, of the American Academy of Acupuncture and Oriental Medicine, explain how imbalance in the Spleen meridian can occur:

> Chinese medicine sees the Spleen as being the key to (the) spiral into fibromyalgia. The Spleen is responsible for transforming the food that we eat into the energy (Chi) and blood that sustain our bodies. Obviously, the health of the Spleen can be affected by inappropriate diet, but it is also strongly affected by the emotion of worry, or over-concentration.
>
> Chronic worry or too much studying eventually interferes with the Spleen's ability to generate and convey sufficient Chi and blood to the muscles and flesh, which is an area of the body that the Spleen is especially responsible for.

Fibromyalgia as a Spiritual Energy Imbalance

The principal muscle that the Spleen needs to sustain is the Heart. The Heart is considered to be the home of the Spirit, and has a close relationship with the Spleen. When the Spleen cannot generate enough substance to nourish the Heart, the Heart Chi does not have enough power to house the spirit properly, and symptoms such as anxiety, palpitations, and insomnia result.

A Spleen Deficiency condition can result in fatigue, muscle stiffness, and pain; a Heart Deficiency condition usually brings emotional unrest and insomnia. These two deficiencies then feed into each other: insomnia causes muscle pain and stiffness, and muscle pain makes sleep more difficult.

The spleen's job is to transform what we eat into nourishment that sustains our body's health. The Spleen meridian can become constricted and weakened when we fall into chronic worry, and the over-concentration of trying to be perfect, a pattern that is typical of the fibromyalgia profile.

You could ask yourself, "Am I burdening myself with toxic materials or thoughts? How am I at breaking down problems into digestible parts? Do I have enough sweetness in my life? Do I have too much sweet in my life?" (Sweets can damage the spleen.)

A person with fibromyalgia probably grew up in a family that fostered a deep need for approval and a powerful expectation of success. When we feel like we must be extremely successful and we need to find our approval outside ourselves, we tighten up inside. We worry that there is something wrong with us, that we won't measure up.

Repeatedly thinking worried, anxious, approval-seeking thoughts can cause constraint in blood vessels and muscles or meridians that deprive the body of essential energy (chi) as well as blood and oxygen. Over time, this constriction can lead to the symptoms of fibromyalgia.

We are tapping on the end of the Spleen meridian when we tap on the point under the arm (four inches below the armpit). This point is Spleen 21. In fact, this point is specifically used for fibromyalgia-type pain.

Tapping for Spleen Meridian Issues

Tap for old beliefs that reflect Spleen energy imbalance:

> *I had to be perfect, or else...*
>
> *I am all alone, I have to do it myself.*
>
> *I have to tough it out and soldier on.*
>
> *I just forge ahead as if nothing is hurting me.*
>
> *I have to pretend everything is okay when I am really feeling lonely or sad.*
>
> *I am sensitive to criticism and I am hard on myself.*
>
> *I worry that I am not doing enough, I'm not good enough.*
>
> *I am really conscientious.*
>
> *When I must compete or be observed while performing a task, I become so nervous and shaky that I do much worse than I would otherwise.*

I am always trying to figure out what everyone else wants instead of I want.

I have to get it right the first time.

The Spleen's positive psycho-emotional attributes are trust, honesty, openness, acceptance, equanimity, balance, and impartiality. We can tap for inviting and choosing and opening into these qualities in our lives.

The Heart Is the Home of the Spirit

Constraint in the Spleen meridian means that it cannot generate enough substance to nourish the Heart, and then the Heart chi does not have enough power to house the spirit properly. Fibromyalgia symptoms such as anxiety and insomnia may appear and eventually show up in the body as fatigue, muscle stiffness, and pain.

Constraint in the Heart, in TCM terms, usually suggests emotional unrest and insomnia. These two deficiencies then feed into each other: insomnia causes muscle pain and stiffness, and muscle pain makes sleep more difficult. Anything that affects the Heart can affect the Spirit.

The Heart meridian begins in the middle of the armpit and flows down the little finger side of the arm, ending at the inside tip of the little finger. The two points on the Heart meridian that we would most likely contact when we tap are: the inside of the little finger; and the wrist on the little finger side just below (i.e., away from the hand) the wrist crease and on the inside of the tendon there. The latter point is called Shen Men/Spirit Gate. In acupuncture, it is utilized specifically for insomnia, anxiety, panic, and mania.

Often when I ask people one of my favorite questions—"Where do you feel that emotion in your body?"—they will say something like "a tightness in my chest," "my heart hurts," "my heart feels heavy." TCM cites one of the Heart meridian's functions as "opens into the tongue." The meridian point Heart 5 is specifically used for the treatment of aphasia—inability to speak.

As spiritual beings, we honor "speaking from the heart" as speaking our own truth.

Tapping for Heart Meridian Issues

Here are some beliefs that reflect a troubled, constricted Heart. As you read them, say each one out loud, while you tap each of the twelve EFT points:

> *I take everything to heart.*
>
> *I don't know how to connect with others without "drowning."*
>
> *I take on everyone else's feelings.*
>
> *I want to please.*
>
> *I so often leave myself last, if I do anything for myself at all.*
>
> *I seem to have trouble saying what I want, especially if I think my preference will hurt someone I care about.*
>
> *I end up keeping quiet and the same pattern continues.*

Fibromyalgia as a Spiritual Energy Imbalance

I feel sad, I feel resentful, I feel depressed and stuck, but I keep my truth inside.

I endlessly worry about what "they" are thinking.

My issue is about not standing up/speaking up for myself.

Connection is more important to me than anything.

I will sell my soul to stay connected.

You might also include these TCM thoughts in your tapping:

Unbalanced Heart energy leads to being careless, forgetful, distracted, restless, and maybe unrealistically idealistic.

Balanced Heart energy is joyful, radiant, outgoing, loving, generous, optimistic, and giving in a grounded way (rather than a giving-myself-away manner).

Move Anger out, Let Your Liver Live!

Sheila, the teacher in our beginning story who experienced the bitter divorce, had a common energy pattern of fibromyalgia, which acupuncturists call "Liver Chi Stagnation."

I am always captured by the name of this organ. Metaphorically, the liver is the part of us that is in charge of our living, the *organizer* of our living fully.

You have probably experienced how anger and fear can interfere with your digestion. I often hear people describe their stomach or their gut as "tied up in knots" when they are upset. If fear, worry, or anger was often present in them in their childhood, but it wasn't safe or considered appropriate for them to express what they felt, they had to swallow what they were feeling. As an adult, all that emotion still sits there in the belly with no place to go.

One of the main functions of the Liver is the smooth flow of chi, blood, and emotions. Extreme or unexpressed anger can compromise its functioning, rendering it "stagnant." We don't want our Liver to be stagnant, either organically or metaphorically! Chinese medicine says that Liver meridian problems "invade" the Spleen or Stomach. This fits with the fact that many people with fibromyalgia—40 to 70 percent, according to one estimate—describe symptoms that are diagnosed by doctors as irritable bowel syndrome. With a lifetime of anger stored in the gut, it is no wonder it gets irritable!

Think of what the digestive system is meant to do—taking in what nourishes us, and letting go of what we no longer need.

Tapping for Liver Meridian Issues

Often as I am tapping with someone whose insides are in a knot of turmoil, I will offer this thought as we tap, perhaps on the Karate Chop point:

Your body knows how to take in, digest, utilize, and release what it no longer needs…. So just let it know that you trust it to process everything that you thought you had to swallow and hang on to…all that anger and fear.

You know instinctively, down deep inside, how to let yourself be nourished by the insights and the knowledge

Fibromyalgia as a Spiritual Energy Imbalance 113

that you have gained from those awful experiences...they have taught you what you don't want, and given you a sense of what you do want instead...so now you are free to move this on through, move it on through now...and let go of what you no longer need.

Your body and your energy system know how to do this...just let that anger and fear go.

The Liver meridian runs from the lateral side of the end of the big toe up the inside of the leg, on both sides of body along the inner part of the ribs. The end point is right under the breast, directly below the nipple, one rib down from the bottom of the breast in both men and women.

EFT tappers seldom utilize this Liver point now, but it is a powerful balancing and harmonizing point for our whole being, and worth including in your tapping round.

Tapping for Small Intestine Meridian Issues

The Small Intestine meridian is paired with the Heart meridian. With long-term stress, such as people with fibromyalgia experience, the Heart can become disturbed and thinking becomes confused. (Long-term stress affects the Spleen first, leading to the Heart disturbance). We become exhausted, breathless, and anxious.

As discussed, the Heart holds the Spirit, the totality of the person's life force as it expresses through the personality. So the physiological function of the Heart energy network, according to TCM, is to propel the blood, enfold the Spirit, and maintain awareness. The Small Intestine meridian's essential purpose is to support our choices about what information to incorporate when we are feeling divided, or pulled in more than one direction. This makes sense when we think of what the small intestine does physiologically. Its job in digestion is to separate what is most useful in the food from what will become waste.

When our system's energy is flowing freely, our Small Intestine protects our Heart by filtering out negative input, both from food waste and damaging energies like shocking surprise or deep sorrow. Even overwhelming joy can be hard on the Heart!

The end point of the Small Intestine energy meridian is on the side of the hand, the Karate Chop point in EFT. (You can also stimulate this meridian by tapping the top, the watch-face side, of either wrist.)

Think about what we are doing when we tap on the side of the hand in EFT. In thought and action, in intention and in energy, we are saying to ourselves:

Even though I have this stressful problem that is upsetting me, I love and accept myself and how I feel anyway.

Even though I am having these stressful experiences, and am telling myself negative things about my self-worth, I understand and appreciate myself anyway, and I am doing the best I can.

There is hope! I value my Spirit. I love that I am making a home for my spirit in my heart.

Summary of Tapping for Fibromyalgia to Bring Harmony to the Spirit

1. Begin with pain in the body.
2. Use imagination and metaphor.
3. Tap for painful experiences.
4. Tap for beliefs that were formed from painful experiences; understand the positive intention.
5. Reframe what happened in a way that nourishes you.
6. Tap for emotions that arise from the constricting beliefs.
7. Tap for self-blame, high expectations, and perfectionism.
8. Invite allowing, opening, grounding, and trusting.
9. Honor sensitivity:

    ...and I honor myself for how hard this has been for me.

    ...and I deserve to take good care of myself.

10. Incorporate your sense of spirituality to build a sense of personal sovereignty:

    This is Where I Stand: I am bringing harmony to my spirit.

Tapping Is "Energy Hygiene"

In his book *Introduction to Incarnational Spirituality*, philosopher and "practical mystic" David Spangler cites the three components of energy hygiene as flow, positivity, and connectedness. He explains:

> Each of us is like a pool of energy. As long as energy is flowing in and out in a healthy way, this pool is alive, clear and clean; when this flow is obstructed by a buildup of "psychic lint," then the pool can begin to stagnate.
>
> Restoring and maintaining a healthy flow of energy is important. A good walk, physical activity, learning something new, doing something kind for someone else are all simple ways of restoring flow; there are also techniques for restoring this flow on a subtle energy level.
>
> Being positive is more than just practicing positive thinking, though that can be helpful. Positivity is a condition of being radiant, open, giving, confident, and strong. It is an energy state as much as a psychological one.
>
> There are many ways of developing and maintaining this state, but they are all enhanced by valuing and honoring yourself and standing in your uniqueness and sovereignty.
>
> Connectedness opens us to a larger world beyond ourselves and enables us to participate in a greater wholeness. A pool stagnates when it is unconnected to living streams of water and ultimately to the ocean

Fibromyalgia as a Spiritual Energy Imbalance 117

on the one hand, and the wellsprings deep within the earth on the other. So too we need to be connected to the vitality and life, the spirit and wellbeing of the world around us.

We create good energy conditions for ourselves not by isolating ourselves behind shields and barriers but by creating good energy in the world around us. Compassionately and lovingly participating in the life of our world and contributing to the wellbeing of all life is a vital part of energy hygiene.*

Healing from Fibromyalgia

Yes, it is possible to heal from fibromyalgia, CFS, Lyme, and autoimmune diseases. And you don't need to know anything about the energy structure of fibromyalgia and the rest of them to be helpful to yourself or others with tapping. However, the language of balancing a person's energy structure is a useful frame in which to hold the story and the healing process.

A spiritual perspective is important. Such a perspective means holding yourself in an honoring, generative, loving way is the taproot and the foundation of transforming yourself from a person who has been diagnosed with fibromyalgia or one of these other conditions into a sacred person.

Engage a deep sense of your birthright to be here, to be you, fully and completely. The opposite of low self-

---

*Reprinted with permission from David Spangler, *Introducion to Incarnational Spirituality*. Everett, WA: Lorian Press, 2011, p. 88.

worth is not self-esteem. It is being fully yourself. It is: *"I deeply and completely love and accept myself, no matter what."*

With EFT and other energy methods we can bring harmony to the energetic patterns of energetic imbalance that Western medicine calls fibromyalgia.

This approach asks us to work with the deepest level of identity. Not everyone is ready for this, but it is a truly worthy road to walk.

Note: For more about Rue Anne Hass and her work, visit www.IntuitiveMentoring.com. For more about tapping for fibromyalgia, click on Books-DVDs/EFT-and-fibromyalgia in the drop-down menu.

Oversight for this article was provided by Charles Chace, DiplAc, DiplCH (http://charleschace.com) and Clariel Hass, LAc.

A good resource for information on fibromyalgia from the perspective of traditional Chinese medicine is *Curing Fibromyalgia Naturally with Chinese Medicine,* by Bob Flaws. See also *The Foundations of Chinese Medicine* and *The Psyche in Chinese Medicine,* both by Giovanni Maciocia.

With appreciation for the ideas and inner awareness of David Spangler, www.lorian.org.

5

The Healing Wave

One of my favorite concepts is that of the healing wave. We saw in some of the earlier examples, such as that of Sarah in chapter 1, that recovery from fibromyalgia, chronic fatigue, and related conditions isn't usually a straight-line path. Patients experience ups and downs in a wavelike pattern. Even though some patients, like Susan in chapter 1, might show dramatic improvement in a single session, the point of using EFT is to maintain you on a lifelong journey of stress release and healing. Here's an example of a straight-line upward path, such as blowing air into a balloon until it is fully inflated, or the temperature of water heated at a constant rate until it boils:

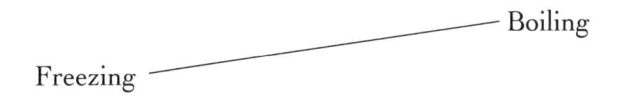

Boiling

Freezing

The healing process is rarely this smooth. It usually occurs in undulating waves. We get a little better, then a little worse, then a little bit even better, then a little bit worse, then better still, then worse, and finally break through our upper limits to become much better. Researcher William Collinge calls this "the healing pattern." The process looks like this:

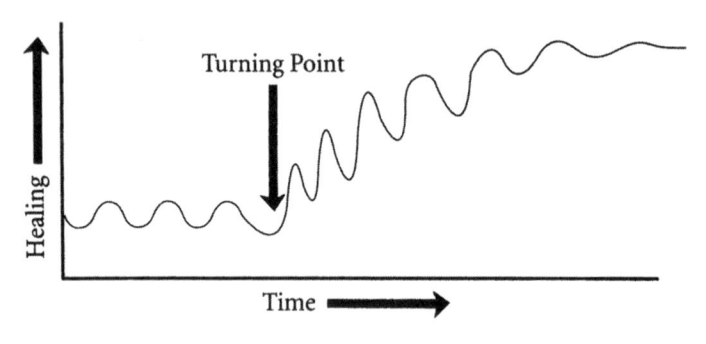

The Healing Pattern

This process is very difficult for you if you're suffering from fibromyalgia, chronic fatigue, or an autoimmune condition. You get a bit better, and this raises your hopes. You think you're on a straight-line upward trend. You may become elated. Then you start getting worse. This apparent reverse makes you feel depressed. You were getting better, now your health has turned back down again. You now imagine you're on a straight-line downward trend.

The Ups and Downs of the Healing Journey

In your reactions to the changes, the fault lies with your thinking and not with your body. If your conscious mind understands the concept of the healing wave, then you understand that every downturn doesn't mean a straight line to doom, and each uptick doesn't mean an inevitable path to immortality. You accept the little ups and downs as steps on the healing journey. The major upward turning point is on one of those waves, and it's usually imperceptible to you at the time it happens. You simply have to stay with the process, riding the waves, mediating your disappointment with EFT, and believing in the possibility that one of those imperceptible shifts marks the turning point. The following story reprinted from EFT Universe, written by Salome Hancock, illustrates that healing wave.

Success Story: EFT on Search-and-Heal Missions

By Salome Hancock

I have had CFIDS (chronic fatigue and immune dysfunction syndrome) for twelve years, and it is a most confounding and disabling disease.

I came across EFT well over a year ago. I watched EFT videos and tapped along with them. I read all the newsletters. I took a Level I EFT weekend training course. I worked a couple of times with an EFT practitioner and went a number of times to an EFT healing circle. Now I work with EFT just about every day on myself and others.

At first, I used it on specific physical symptoms and experienced relief and help, which greatly encouraged me to continue. I have been absolutely amazed by how much EFT helps with the many

CFIDS symptoms that continuously arise. I could list a pageful of physical symptoms that I cycle through. Time and again, EFT would diminish or neutralize symptoms such as nausea, pain, foggy brain, aches, crash from overexertion, reaction to being out in sun and wind, skin reactions, plus many more.

CFIDS is a complex and deep-seated condition. It was hard to budge this massive problem, which had settled in and taken over every aspect and level of my being (physical, mental, psychological, spiritual). At my worst, I stayed in bed and couldn't tolerate light or activity, only accomplishing the most basic maintenance. Going out, seeing people, and being involved in activities were impossible when I was at my worst.

As I used EFT, experienced its help, and gained confidence in it, I started taking it deeper. I worked with visualization and metaphor, which seemed to get me closer to the roots of my illness. For example, when I work with EFT, I picture obstacles being removed and the energy flowing freely through my system. I "see" the energy moving around. I "send" it to damaged areas and ask it to do repair work. I send the healing forces on search missions to find broken parts—from the distant past and from the present—and I give the energies time to bring in whatever is needed for that site. I express confidence that problems found are being worked on.

I "installed" an optimum wellness computer program in the foundation of my being. Ever since, I bring whatever is needed on a particular day to "reboot" and make any corrections and connections necessary to help me improve function and well-being for that day. I went back with all the forces I could summon to painful things that had happened to me—sources of grief, rage, unfairness—and concentrated energies on repairing, on bringing all parts of my being into alignment to support my progress back to health.

I revisited times and events that caused me to give up in despair, and brought healing energy to whatever it was. I brought love, compassion, and forgiveness, for myself in not being able to cope, and for those who injured me.

I am not cured, but friends have noticed that I have increased ability to function, more sustained energy, and more discipline in how I approach my goals. I notice stretches of much-improved functioning. My brain is working better. I've turned around the atrophy that was creeping over me. I am exercising now. I had concluded with absolute conviction that exercise was out of the question for me ever again. I opened myself up to its possibility with perseverance and the help of EFT. I'm gaining strength now; I can see and feel it. I am pursuing painting as never before. I am in an exciting process of discovery now and feel hope that *I can get better, and will keep getting better,* and am thoroughly open to these possibilities.

❉ ❉ ❉

Like Salome, you can use EFT to remove obstacles to your healing. Perhaps we should all take a tip from her and look at the exploration of the roots of our illness and of what is stopping us from getting well as "an exciting process of discovery." When you're on that downward slope in the healing spiral, it's easy to lose sight of your progress.

One of the most common issues observed in patients with fibromyalgia and chronic fatigue is a sense of hopelessness. They've felt bad for so long, they have little belief that they might get better. EFT Master Practitioner Maggie Adkins calls this the "Why Bother" syndrome. Why try something new when you've tried dozens of other remedies and none of them has been successful? Each new approach has raised your hopes, which have then been dashed when it proves as fleeting as the last. This leads to hopelessness, a state in which you don't try new remedies because your track record of failure predisposes you to believe that the next possible approach is going to lead you on the same cycle of hope and despair as the previous approaches have yielded. In the following essay, Maggie talks about this problem, and ways to overcome it.

The "Why Bother" Syndrome

By Maggie Adkins, EFT Master Practitioner

One of the more subtle challenges that gets in the way of people using EFT is when they have already worked on issues and emotions "ad nauseam" (as one client says) with other therapies over the years, and yet these issues have not lessened or been released. Intellectually, we may know that EFT is different from other therapies, and still we listen to our minds saying, "Why bother? Nothing is going to change this."

"Why Bother" stops many of us from the success we could have if we used EFT to release old issues, drop those cravings, and shift that negative belief. Because EFT is most effective when we are tapping on the correct issue, "Why Bother" can truly sabotage our EFT results.

The first problem is that we may not do EFT at all. The essence of "Why Bother" is that it isn't going to make a difference anyway so why would we do EFT? "It's just a waste of time," the mind says. That's not much motivation to do the work.

The second problem is that we may be tapping on what we think is the issue, but the real issue we have to clear first is "Why Bother."

"Why Bother" usually takes the form of resistance to "one more therapy that's supposed to help, " or uncovering that issue "one more time." If you hear your mind saying, "I'm all right. I can cope," that is also a form of "Why Bother." To say you have to cope is to say that you have given up, that you don't believe the problem can be released. I hear many clients say this as we go from a 10 to a 2 or 3 on the intensity meter. I ask them, "If we have gotten this down to a 2 or 3, why not see if we can just get rid of it? I don't know if we can, but why not go for it?" It's a good question.

Examples of "Why Bother" Thoughts

Here are some typical examples of what you might think if you have "Why Bother." Are any of these voices in your head?

- For attempting something that didn't go well in the past: *"Why would I want to try that again? Look what happened the other times! It was a disaster."*

- For weight loss: *"I've lost 300 pounds in my life—and gained back 310. If I drop weight, I'll just gain it back and hate myself all over again—why bother?"*

- For relationship issues: *"You want me in a loving relationship with a significant other? Risk loving again? I'd rather stay safe and just cope with my own little life. I refuse to open myself up again just to be hurt. No way am I going through that one again!"*

- For chronic fatigue, environmental illness, and other chronic conditions: *"You don't know how many people have said they could help me and none of them have. I'm not putting myself through that again. It's just too disappointing."*

- For business owners (EFT practitioners included, of course): *"Look, I already sent out all those flyers and newsletters and everyone knows I'm in business. I'm not going through all that expense and heartache again when people don't call. I'm probably just not good enough anyway."*

- For posttraumatic stress disorder (PTSD): *"Yeah, right. Do you know how many people have said they can help these Vietnam memories over the last forty years? Well, I used to listen to them but no more. I am not going into that stuff again. It's just too hard."*

If you have any of these voices in your mind, you probably have resistance to doing EFT—and yet, EFT can shift all that.

How Do I Heal This?

These negative voices in the mind take away motivation to actually do the EFT that can release the issue/pain/negative belief. They can also drain self-esteem: "I must be a failure because nothing has worked for me."

My good friend and skilled EFT practitioner Mary Ann Michels makes the excellent suggestion that you first write down all the "Why Bother" thoughts you are conscious of thinking. I find that making a list can, indeed, help a great deal when working with this kind of issue. You can make an initial list and, as you tap on one or more of those thoughts, you may find that even more sabotaging thoughts come into your consciousness. Stop what you're doing and write them down! This is one of the miracles of the EFT journey. It simply seems to take us where we are to go. I would keep paper and pen handy when doing this work. (And thank you, Mary Ann, for your valuable insights.)

If you do make a list, each time you begin an EFT session with yourself, ask yourself which thought is the most powerful right now. Doing EFT with the issue that is most intense can often provide the greatest healing.

Sample EFT Phrases for "Why Bother"

The goal is to acknowledge all the reasons you don't want to do EFT and tap for those very thoughts, as much as possible in your own words. Here are just a few examples of how to use EFT for "Why Bother":

Sample Setup Statement (say this three times while tapping on the Karate Chop Point or rubbing the Sore Spot on the chest): *"Even though I have done everything I could think of to heal this before and it didn't work, and now I don't believe anything can heal this, I deeply and profoundly accept myself."*

Sample Reminder Phrase (say this while tapping through all the other EFT points): *"Nothing can heal this. Why bother?"*

You can say the Reminder Phrase at each point or you can alternate it with "Why bother?" If you alternate, it might be something like this:

Top of Head: *Nothing can heal this.*

Eyebrow: *Why bother?*

Side of Eye: *Nothing can heal this.*

Under Eye: *Why bother?*

Under Nose: *Nothing can heal this.*

Chin: *Why bother?*

Collarbone: *Nothing can heal this.*

Under Arm: *Why bother?*

Sample Setup: *"Even though I have attempted many times to get rid of these emotions, they're still here. I don't know if they'll ever go away, and I deeply and profoundly accept myself."*

Sample Reminder Phrase: *"Nothing worked. Why should this be different?"*

Again, you can say the Reminder Phrases at each point or you can alternate.

Sample Setup: *"Even though I have attempted to get rid of this pain time and time again with much heavier therapies than EFT and it's still here, I deeply and profoundly accept myself. I'm terrified (or afraid) that it will never go away."*

Sample Reminder Phrase: *"Already tried to get rid of it and it's still here. Terrified (or afraid) it might never go away."*

Sample Setup: *"Even though I've done my best to get rid of this [name what "this" is; be as specific as possible] and it's still here, I deeply and profoundly accept myself. I'm afraid it will get worse, my body is so out of control. I deeply and profoundly accept myself anyway. And I accept that sometimes I don't accept myself."*

Sample Reminder Phrase: *"Done my best and it's still here. Body is sooo out of control and I'm afraid it will get worse."*

Sample Setup: *"Even though I am so afraid to love again, maybe I have learned some things, maybe it doesn't have to be the same way again, and again, I deeply and profoundly accept myself."*

Sample Reminder Phrase: *"So afraid, so afraid, so afraid to love." "Maybe I've learned—maybe it can be better. Maybe—maybe not."*

Sample Setup: *"Even though I'm terrified to go into this again—nothing else has worked, why would EFT work, I deeply and profoundly accept myself."*

Sample Reminder Phrase: *"Terrified to go into this again. Nothing else has worked—why would EFT work?"*

Sample Setup: *"Even though I'm terrified to quit my day job and just go for it, I deeply and profoundly accept myself. Other people are full time EFTers—why can't I do it?"*

Sample Reminder Phrase: *"Terrified to quit my day job and go for it. Others do it, what's wrong with me?"*

This is also a good time to use "parts" EFT. With this technique, you address both parts of yourself in the same EFT round. You address the part that wants to heal and the part that is afraid to heal or for some reason doesn't want to heal. Instead of separate rounds, you combine them, which is often very powerful. Please incorporate your own words whenever you can. Here is a generic example:

Sample Setup: *"Even though a part of me wants to release this, a part of me is terrified to go there again and feel all those feelings. I deeply and profoundly accept myself anyway."*

You might want to alternate this Reminder Phrase even if you haven't done so before: *"Part of me is terrified. Part of me wants to heal."*

The Healing Wave   131

Adding Forgiveness

After doing several rounds of EFT, you might want to introduce forgiveness. The timing of this is individual and you can use your intuition to know when to add it. You might say something like:

"I forgive myself for any contribution I may have made to this problem/issue/whatever you want to call it."

You can expand forgiveness to include something like:

"I forgive whoever may have played a part in this."

If you believe in God, you might add:

"I forgive whoever may have played a part in this, including God."

Add the forgiveness phrases wherever you want. You can add them as a part of the Setup Statement or at any or all of the rest of the EFT points.

Specific Traumas or Issues

Doing this work will most probably lead you back to the specific events or traumas that you wanted to heal in the first place. Remember, attempting to heal them in the past is probably why you have the "Why Bother" Syndrome. Start by working with your "Why Bother" phrases and see where they lead you. As you release "Why Bother," you can then do EFT with much more motivation on those issues and problems that you wanted to heal to begin with.

Shifting Your Old Conditioning

If you have the "Why Bother" Syndrome, and you are still reading this, it may be time to take the chance and see for yourself if EFT can shift those old conditionings. Of course, we base our truths on past experience. With the arrival of EFT, however, so much has changed that it is not valid anymore to give up and say, "This is just the way it is. It is too big for me to change."

We can now take those issues and problems that we thought we had to "cope" with and simply do EFT. Chances are we can do a lot more than cope. Chances are we can release the chains to our past and move toward our Palace of Possibilities. If you are not familiar with Palace of Possibilities, please see EFT's website (www.EFTuniverse.com) for an extensive manuscript on using EFT for positive affirmations.

As with all issues, there are times when it is helpful to seek a professional practitioner. Most EFT practitioners I know do telephone consultations daily, so geography need not play a role in your choice of a practitioner. About 95 percent of my current clients work with me via phone consultations; I have clients in both the United States and Australia. In my experience, these work as well as in-person consultations. One telephone client in the United States said recently, "I didn't know intuition could fly halfway around the world. This is great!"

My Journey out of Fibromyalgia with EFT

By Kristina Lukawska

A year ago, on Christmas Eve, I started to experience severe pain in my joints and muscles. They were heavy flu-like symptoms. After a few weeks of constant pain, I went to a doctor and I was diagnosed with fibromyalgia.

I was in pain almost all the time. I had a few good days followed by a few bad weeks. I used to be a very active person, rarely watching TV. Suddenly I came back home from work, often early, and I spent the rest of the day in bed watching TV or sleeping.

Even worse than the pain was fatigue. It was nothing like normal fatigue. I often had problems walking; each step needed conscious extra effort from me. At times lifting my arm or leg was like lifting heavy weights. I stopped doing many things automatically. Many activities, even really small ones, like getting a cup out from a shelf, needed special effort. I could be exhausted after brushing my teeth even though I washed them sitting down. I had difficulties putting on my clothes. It was such a challenge to get ready for work in the morning. I felt like I was a hundred years old.

I felt embarrassed; I did not know how to talk about it with my family and friends. I was probably afraid that they might tell me that I am overreacting, that it's all in my head. I started to go to different alternative practitioners and they kept telling me that I have chosen my fibromyalgia. It did not help; it just made me feel guilty. I tried different diets including fasting and I had some relief but after a while the pain and fatigue would always return.

Around May, a friend of mine told me about EFT. I printed the manual from the web site and I signed up for a upcoming seminar. I went to a three day seminar in Chicago and my intuition told me that this was going to be the method for me. The most attractive part was the fact that I could do it myself, that I didn't feel powerless. At the seminar I met Andy Bryce and I asked him to work with me. He seemed like a very considerate and compassionate, gentle person. He has been working with me over the phone for the past five months and my life has changed amazingly.

Even though the whole process, which brought me to the moment where I am now, is important, there are a few steps that I feel are particularly worth mentioning (stepping stones).

The first one was the session when Andy sent me his love energy and helped me experience the love. It was the first time I was completely freed of pain. It gave me strength and faith that I could be healed. After that I noticed a big shift in my energy. I stopped being fatigued most of the time. I also noticed that it was getting much easier to listen to my intuition.

Next, we began work on my core issue, which was my guilt, and sense of responsibility for my mother's suffering, and the belief that "I must suffer in my life." So Andy suggested to tap on, "I believe that I must suffer a lot in my life" and, "I didn't deserve to be healthy and happy" and, "I don't believe I can free myself from suffering." I also tapped a lot for affirmations like, "I'm willing to open my heart to myself" and, "I love being healthy." Especially important for me was "I'm grateful for this pain gift which brought me understanding and compassion but I'm willing to learn from joy." I also tapped on experiences from my past associated with this.

At the end of September, when I was at a Buddhist retreat, I started to feel a sharp pain under my left shoulder. After a while, the pain became more and more nagging. Since I have had fibromyalgia my sleep was shallow, especially in the mornings, after 2 to 3 am. So, now, with this new pain, I woke up dozens of times throughout the night. I was growing increasingly frustrated; I was tired and desperate to get some sleep. The more I tried to resist the pain, the more it persisted. I woke up every hour to struggle with the pain. I started to tap on, "I'm willing to receive the message that the pain gives me." After a while I found out that I needed this pain; I sometimes greet it with gratitude. I almost enjoyed my wakeful nights; it helps me practice holding my attention on my breath. And again Andy suggested to tap on, " "I'm grateful for the message this pain gives me and I recognize the fear behind it but I'm willing to see if my path to enlightenment can be filled with joy and gratefulness."

In November I went to Toronto for the Energy Psychology Conference. I attended the workshop led by Steven Vazquez and for a moment I was freed of the pain while the presenter was working with somebody suffering from fibromyalgia. Completely intuitively I asked Steven for a private session.

At the session I asked him to work on my specific back pain. We reconstructed the lineage from which the pain had come. The links brought me through the retreat and suffering to my childhood, World War II, my parents and my mother's depression. A few times he asked me to stand up and kept his hands hovering inches away from my body while we were talking. We spent some time talking about my mother's suffering. I wanted to free her from her pain and misery. The pain under my shoulder was getting more intense. He asked me to I give my mother back all the hurt in a symbolic way. I did it and I felt an enormous relief.

A few moments after that I felt immense happiness. I started to laugh and I laughed with all my heart. I stopped laughing as I felt this huge wave of joy coming toward me. I felt like the gate to the Universe had opened. I saw two different spaces. I felt I was in both spaces. I felt pain in my back but it felt very different. It did not bother me at all. It was just something I once called pain. I was completely free of hurt. Everything seemed to be lucid and transparent.

After a while I felt an even deeper wave of joy. I felt an amazing hoop vibrating around my heart. This new space had opened up for me and I felt infinitely and entirely free and complete. I did not feel joy, I was joy. And everything else was joy. There was nothing before or beyond. There was no time. There

The Healing Wave 137

was pure and absolutely perfect joy. Then gratitude emerged and I was so very grateful to Steven who was sitting in front of me. I hugged him and I felt profound gratitude to all sentient beings, to my teachers and my family, my neighbors and all the people I used to be afraid of. It was endless gratitude.

My session was over and I returned to the conference. For the next few days I was filled with blissful joy. I felt such amazing lightness in my body. The pain began to vanish and each day there was less and less of it. After a couple days I slept through the whole night with no pain. After ten days I was completely freed of the pain.

My life has changed dramatically. I am freed of my past. Now Andy helps me work to create the future I want. I would like to be an EFT therapist and trainer.

I am deeply grateful to Andy Bryce for improving the quality of my life, relieving my pain, and helping me become more compassionate towards other people as well as myself, helping me be more receptive to my intuition. I am NOT a victim of fibromyalgia anymore. I took ownership for whatever has happen in my life. I experience pain at some level but it doesn't bother me. I know that I can take good care of myself and I am going to be completely healed.

I am profoundly grateful for helping me to open the gate to my new life—a life full of adventures, surprises, love, joy, connections, and responsibility without guilt.

※ ※ ※

Isn't this a wonderful story? I trust that you feel great hope as you read it. Imagine that what you've just read isn't Kristina's story; it's your story. Imagine that in a few weeks, you're emailing your story of healing from fibromyalgia to the EFT newsletter editor for publication and sharing with others, just the way Kristina and the other people in this book have done. The fact that they made this progress demonstrates that it's really possible, and that the next miracle just might be you.

Persisting Through the Cycles

In this chapter, we've reviewed the concept of the healing cycle. If you weren't aware of this phenomenon, you might become needlessly depressed when faced with minor and temporary setbacks in your heath. You might also become unreasonably elated at minor and temporary improvements. If you're aware that both of these patterns are small brushstrokes in a bigger picture, and that the pivotal point of healing happens imperceptibly, my hope is that you'll be encouraged to persevere on your healing journey. You won't be fazed by the little downturns; you won't attach great weight to upticks. Instead, you will, as Rudyard Kipling advised, "meet with triumph and disaster, and treat those two impostors just the same." This gives you a huge amount of freedom—you can keep plugging away at the EFT routine throughout the entire span of your healing process.

6

Moving Forward

You now have all the information you need about how EFT can help you heal from fibromyalgia and chronic fatigue, as well as Lyme and other autoimmune diseases. It only remains for you to build tapping into your life so you can begin to watch your symptoms decrease and take your first steps toward living free of pain and exhaustion. With what you know already, you are equipped to start integrating EFT into your everyday routines. The tapping scripts you experienced in chapters 1 and 3 are enough to get you going.

You can use daily tapping on whatever issues arise for you, as they arise. You can also use EFT's Personal Peace Procedure (as described in chapter 2) to systematically clear all the traumas from your past, which you have been carrying around with you all these years and which are likely contributing to your health problems, perhaps profoundly. Following either of these routes will produce positive—or even miraculous—effects on your health.

You may, however, prefer more guidance. There is a wealth of tapping guidance available to you from a range of sources: EFTuniverse.com, DVDs, EFT practitioners, tapping groups, and, most specific to your health condition, the online program that serves as a companion to this book—the *EFT 12-Week Program for Fibromyalgia and Chronic Fatigue* (www.FibroClear.com). In the twelve weeks of this detailed program, you will tap through the challenges most frequently associated with fibromyalgia and chronic fatigue.

The following are some of the most common challenges that people with fibromyalgia and chronic fatigue face. The FibroClear program (www.FibroClear.com) takes you through specific EFT protocols to address each of these challenges in turn.

Pain Reduction

Vital to reducing your pain is gaining a complete understanding of the what, where, and when of your pain: What increases or triggers your pain? Where in your body is your pain focused? When in the day or night is your pain at its worst? The answers to these questions comprise your pain profile, which provides you with a road map for reducing your pain. When you know the factors that contribute to the pain, you can take steps to reduce or avoid those factors and schedule your activity for your best times of day. By managing your pain, you halt the downward spiral of pain and exhaustion, as each compounds the other. Your pain profile will also guide you in the timing and focus of your tapping for pain reduction.

Self-care is another important tool in reducing your pain. To provide effective self-care, you need to look at all the areas of your life—work, relationships, finances, physical exercise, diet, relaxation, and fun—and consider which ones are lacking balance. Which areas are you neglecting or overdoing? Which could use nurturing?

Here is a quote from one of the success stories of reducing fibromyalgia pain with EFT: "Mum feels so much better that she is now considering at some point in the future joining a gym for some gentle exercise. She has also not required any of her daily painkillers for forty-eight hours and counting. This is a massive breakthrough, as prior to doing EFT, her mindset was one of 'I can't cope without my co-codamol' and 'I'm never going to get over this.' Now, as she says in her own words, 'I can now see light at the end of the tunnel.'"

Stress and Emotional Upset

There is a strong association between high stress levels and fibromyalgia/CFS. Studies have demonstrated that when patients improve their stress levels, their physical symptoms improve as well. People with fibromyalgia and chronic fatigue often have psychological conditions such as anxiety, depression, and posttraumatic stress disorder. Stress can exacerbate these conditions as well as your pain and fatigue.

You may not be able to change the circumstances of your daily life, but you can change your reactions to those circumstances. Emotional upset is a stress reaction and raises your overall stress level. Tapping on your emotional upset can help you manage your stress and reduce the psychological and physical symptoms of your illness.

Think about the emotional reactions you had over the past several weeks. Are they clustered in one or several areas of your life—work, family, other relationships, finances, or health? Where is your biggest cluster? The area where your emotional reactions are most concentrated gives you a clue as to what emotional issue to tap on first.

Sue, who suffered from fibromyalgia, tapped on the emotions connected to a car accident that had occurred twelve years before. Here's what happened after EFT: All Sue could do was laugh. She said she felt so light and happy. What a relief to lay down a pain she had carried for twelve years. Checking in one month later, Sue said that she has had no shoulder pain and that her life is changing for the better every day.

Past Trauma

As discussed throughout this book, the reason that certain people or situations bother you today is almost always because they remind your brain of a similar situation that occurred early in your life. Childhood traumas are like templates. When a current event fits the template, your brain's stress machinery springs to life. Unless you reduce the emotional intensity of the childhood memory, you will continue to respond with emotional upset to events in the present.

Old childhood memories may even be at the root of your fibromyalgia and chronic fatigue itself. According to the National Institutes of Health, "Many people associate the development of fibromyalgia with a physically or emotionally stressful or traumatic event, such as an automobile accident." Best-selling author and natural health advocate Joseph Mercola, DO, has discovered the same in his medical practice: "In my experience fibromyalgia is nearly always related to some severe emotional trauma that establishes a series of potentially devastating physical processes, which frequently incapacitate the person."

Looking for childhood templates for current upsets and tapping on those childhood memories to heal them can improve or even resolve your fibromyalgia and chronic fatigue.

In another fibromyalgia success story, after tapping on an intense emotional memory, Sharon was enjoying her thirteenth night and counting of falling asleep without pain. "This is a phenomenal record for me," she said. Her days were free of pain as well.

Hopelessness and Helplessness

Living with the limitations that a chronic illness imposes is highly frustrating, to say the least! It often raises feelings of hopelessness about the future and helplessness in the face of the accompanying physical restrictions and medical needs and procedures. As you become increasingly pessimistic about the future and your prognosis, it is easy to fall into a disaster mentality, a tendency to catastrophize everything, for example, "Oh no, my leg is hurting. It's going to get so bad that I won't be able to walk and I'll have to be in a wheelchair for the rest of my life." Catastrophizing can cause you to limit your physical movement and effort more than you need to as you anticipate that the worst will happen. In response, your sense of hopelessness and helplessness increases. With EFT, you can extricate yourself from this vicious cycle. Research demonstrates that EFT can reduce anxiety and "pain catastrophizing measures" (helplessness, rumination, and magnification) in people with fibromyalgia.

When tuning into the thoughts running through their brains, most people are surprised to discover how many of these thoughts are negative. Examples of this negative self-talk are "I'll never be healthy" or "Pain is my middle name" or "What's the use?" Even without you tuning in, such negative thoughts about yourself and your situation exert their negative effects on your physical, emotional, and spiritual well-being. Your negative self-talk feeds your sense of helplessness and hopelessness.

Tapping directly on the feelings of helplessness and hopelessness will leave you feeling more positive. EFT can also help you reverse your negative self-talk, so it no longer undermines your health.

Low Self-Esteem

When you are chronically ill, it's difficult not to begin to suffer from low self-esteem. You may not be able to engage in the activities from which you used to derive a sense of accomplishment, and the roles on which you used to base your identity may now be severely limited or even gone. As with the other challenges discussed here, a vicious cycle is often set in motion: feeling bad about yourself results in you limiting your activity, which in turn worsens your self-image, which leads to doing less, and so on.

Many of the symptoms and emotions associated with fibromyalgia and chronic fatigue are also signs of low self-esteem, including anxiety, depression, fear, shame, guilt, and focus on your limits (or what you perceive to be your limits). Another vicious circle is created: the lower your self-image, the easier it is to get upset and the more intense become your emotional responses.

You can actually tap for self-esteem and, as noted previously, tap away your negative self-talk, a big contributor to poor self-image. Improving your view of yourself is vital to healing. With healthy self-esteem, you are more resilient and better able to weather stress and setbacks, and less likely to experience feelings such as hopelessness, worthlessness, guilt, and shame.

In the success story of another fibromyalgia sufferer, one of Lisette's stepping-stones was the work she did on her core issue: her guilt and responsibility for her mother's suffering with the attendant belief "I must suffer in my life." Her EFT practitioner suggested that Lisette tap on: "I believe that I must suffer a lot in my life" and "I don't deserve to be healthy and happy." She also tapped frequently on the affirmations "I'm willing to open my heart to myself" and "I love being healthy." Now she says, "I am not a victim of fibromyalgia anymore. I took ownership for whatever happened in my life. I experience pain at some level, but it doesn't bother me. I know that I can take good care of myself and I am going to be completely healed."

Secondary Gain

Sometimes there are benefits in keeping an illness, detrimental behaviors, and negative thoughts in place. These benefits, known as secondary gain, may be blocking you from getting better. And you may not even be aware of them.

A common secondary gain is the benefit to be had from victimhood. Being a victim gives you a certain status and earns you a lot of attention. If you got well, you might lose that attention. Other examples of secondary gain in the case of fibromyalgia and chronic fatigue might be the constant companionship of caregivers, help from friends and family, disability compensation, or the ability to keep denying the original cause of the pain.

If you do not first clear the obstacles to your healing—your subconscious attachments to being ill—tapping on your pain, other symptoms, or emotional issues associated with your illness may not be effective. You need to clear the blockage to allow tapping to work optimally. To accomplish this, EFT can help you uncover the direct and indirect benefits you receive from being ill. Keep in mind during this process, however, that just because a part of you appreciates some benefits from being ill doesn't mean another part of you doesn't want to get well. Leaving victimhood behind doesn't mean blaming the victim. Be gentle and kind to yourself.

Significant healing work occurs outside as well as within your tapping scripts. The self-inquiry process that gives you specific material for tapping is as important as the tapping. There is much to learn from turning within and exploring all aspects of your illness.

Once you've identified how your illness serves you, you can tap on those secondary gains and dispel them, which removes obstacles to your healing.

Fears about Your Future

Fear is another obstacle to healing. Fear about the future is understandably one of the most common fears among fibromyalgia and chronic fatigue sufferers, as in "I'm afraid that I'll never be well again" or "I'm afraid that I'll be in this terrible pain forever." In order to envision the best that you can be, you will need to tap away your fear. Then the images of what you really want and all the possibilities awaiting you can emerge.

You can use the process of self-inquiry to make a list of your fears about the future. The nature of fear is that it loses some of its hold on you when you state it out loud or write it down on paper. The more you state your fear or look at it, the less potent it becomes. Fear likes the dark. Making a list shines some light on your fears and helps dispel them. Tapping does the rest. You can tap through your list of fears and then tap on other fears about the future, as they arise.

Paula's symptoms at first disappeared with EFT, but then: "After a couple of weeks, some of the fibromyalgia symptoms started to reappear. I started to get worried [fear of the future], so I contacted Clay [her EFT practitioner]. He wanted me to know that just because some symptoms started to return, it didn't mean that EFT hadn't worked for me. It was simply that more issues from my past needed to be addressed. So, over the next few months, I resolved these issues. Once again, my symptoms disappeared."

Accepting the Unacceptable

How can we make peace with having fibromyalgia and chronic fatigue, or with having undergone terrible traumas? It is about "accepting the unacceptable," says Swedish researcher Gunilla Brattberg, MD, authority on fibromyalgia and CFS. There are strategies you can use to facilitate acceptance. These include some of the approaches to the challenges we're discussing here, such as stress and pain management, letting go of victimhood, and processing trauma. And you can tap directly on accepting the unacceptable and tap away "unforgivable" events.

One person with fibromyalgia said she felt she had let God down by being so ill that she could not do the work she was supposed to do. She tapped on: "I accept myself even though I have this disease." The pain in both arms disappeared immediately!

The Mother Wound

Some of the emotional traumas stored within you come from events or incidents involving your mother or another important female figure from your childhood, such as a grandmother, sister, aunt, or teacher. There are many kinds of wounding. The very person you most needed care from might have neglected or abused you. You may have lost your mother at a young age. You may have been given up for adoption. Your mother may have shamed, ridiculed, or criticized you. Your mother may have been sweet and loving most of the time but criticized you in a moment of frustration or impatience that had nothing to do with you. That event may have left a wound that causes you to react in the present to a person or circumstance that your brain sees as similar to the wounding experience with your mother—that childhood template again.

An unresolved mother wound can underlie a wide range of physical and psychological ailments. Though you may not be able to draw a causal link between your fibromyalgia/CFS and stored trauma relating to your mother, you only increase your chances of reducing your pain and fatigue by tapping away the upset that produces tension, depletes your energy, and negatively impacts how you look at the world and yourself.

In Barbara's success story, the morning after she tapped away crucial wounding events associated with her mother, all of her fibromyalgia pain was gone, or maybe at a rating of 1, and it has not returned. She was sleeping better, was able to work more, her nose was less runny, and her irritable bowel syndrome was mostly gone.

The Father Wound

As with the mother wound, there are many kinds of wounding associated with fathers or other significant males from your childhood. Your wound may have involved abuse, a physically absent or emotionally distant father, a longing for approval never received, or shaming and ridicule. A common form of the father wound is from the angry, authoritarian father. The wounding from the anger, which is terrifying to a child (made even more frightening by the physical size of the father, often much bigger and stronger than the child's mother), has far-reaching effects. Growing up in fear produces fearful adults with low self-esteem.

Like an unhealed mother wound, an unresolved father wound can contribute to or exacerbate a wide range of physical and psychological problems. In addition, as long as you carry that father wound, your ability to approach the world in the present, instead of as a reaction to the past, is compromised. You can tap to heal your father wound and tap to heal father issues as they arise.

An EFT practitioner reports the successful resolution of a cluster of fears related to Josie's alcoholic "monster uncle": "I am still astounded when I think about how easy it was to clear her affliction with fibromyalgia pain throughout her whole body, which she had suffered from for so many years. Who would have known or ever expected that fibromyalgia could have been related to fear of spiders, men, monsters, or alcoholics?"

Creating a Positive Future

Perhaps the biggest challenge faced by people with fibromyalgia and chronic fatigue is belief in a positive future. In the midst of pain and exhaustion, among a range of other symptoms, it's difficult to believe that you will ever get better, much less be able to live your dreams. By the time you reach the end of the *EFT 12-Week Program for Fibromyalgia and Chronic Fatigue* (www.FibroClear.com), you will have cleared many of the obstacles that prevented you from believing in a positive future. You will have addressed all of the challenges we've discussed here and you will be feeling much better on all levels—physically, mentally, emotionally, and spiritually. You will have freed yourself to dream big and tap on your vision. Tapping on a powerful image creates an emotional charge that will catalyze positive change. As with other tapping statements, the more specific you can be, the better the outcome. So dream big and dream in detail. The workbook will guide you through creating your vision of a positive future and then tapping to catalyze your new life.

❊ ❊ ❊

When you have fibromyalgia, chronic fatigue, Lyme disease, or another autoimmune disorder, the challenges facing you often feel overwhelming. Being in pain and exhausted makes the challenges even more formidable. EFT is a simple, practical way to begin healing. You can tap when you are in pain. You can tap when you are exhausted. You can tap when you are afraid. You can tap when you feel hopeless. In other words, you can tap anytime and for everything! As your symptoms begin to improve or even disappear, the challenges facing you become less daunting. You know you have a technique that can help you meet any challenge that arises. You have a technique to help you move through that challenge, often quickly. With what you have learned in this book, you have everything you need to begin healing right now.

May you soon be free of pain and fatigue!

EFT Glossary

The following terms have specific meanings in EFT. They are referred to in some of the reports included here and are often mentioned in EFT reports.

Acupoints. Acupuncture points that are sensitive points along the body's meridians. Acupoints can be stimulated by acupuncture needles or, in acupressure, by massage or tapping. EFT is an acupressure tapping technique.

Art of Delivery. The sophisticated presentation of EFT that uses imagination, intuition, and humor to quickly discover and treat the underlying causes of pain and other problems. The art of delivery goes far beyond basic EFT.

Aspects. "Issues within issues," or different facets or pieces of a problem that are related but separate. When new aspects appear, EFT can seem to stop working. In truth, the original EFT treatment continues to work while the new aspect triggers a new set of symptoms. In some cases, many aspects of a situation or problem each require their own EFT treatment. In others, only a few do.

Basic Recipe (also known as Mechanical EFT). EFT's basic protocol, which consists of tapping on the Karate Chop point or Sore Spot while saying three times, "Even though I have this __[problem]__, I fully and complete accept myself" (Setup Phrase), followed by three rounds of tapping the Sequence of EFT acupoints in order, with an appropriate Reminder Phrase. See also Full Basic Recipe.

Borrowing Benefits. When you tap with or on behalf of another person, your own situation improves, even though you aren't tapping for your own situation. This happens in one-on-one sessions, in groups, and when you perform surrogate or proxy tapping. The more you tap for others, the more your own life improves.

Chasing the Pain. After applying EFT, physical discomforts can move to other locations and/or change in intensity or quality. A headache described as a sharp pain behind the eyes at an intensity of 8 might shift to a dull throb at the back of the head at an intensity of 7 (or 9, or 3, or any other intensity level). Moving pain is an indication that EFT is working. Keep "chasing the pain" with EFT and it will usually go to 0 or some low number. In the process, emotional issues behind the discomforts are often successfully treated.

Chi. Vital energy that flows through and around every living being. Chi is said to regulate spiritual, emotional, mental, and physical balance and to be influenced by *yin* (the receptive, feminine force) and *yang* (the active masculine force). These forces, which are complementary opposites, are in constant motion. When yin and yang are balanced, they work together with the natural flow of chi

EFT Glossary

to help the body achieve and maintain health. Chi moves through the body along invisible pathways, or channels, called meridians. Traditional Chinese medicine identifies twenty meridians through which chi flows or circulates to all parts of the body. Acupoints along the meridians can be stimulated to improve the flow of chi and, in EFT, to resolve emotional issues.

Choices Method. Dr. Patricia Carrington's method for inserting positive statements and solutions into Setup and Reminder Phrases.

Core Issues. Deep, important underlying emotional imbalances, usually created in response to traumatic events. A core issue is truly the crux of the problem, its root or heart. Core issues are not always obvious but careful detective work can often uncover them and, once discovered, they can be broken down into specific events and handled routinely with EFT.

Full Basic Recipe. A four-step treatment consisting of Setup phrase, Sequence (tapping on acupoints in order), 9-Gamut Procedure, and Sequence. This was the original EFT protocol.

Generalization Effect. When related issues are neutralized with EFT, they often take with them issues that are related in the person's mind. In this way, several issues can be resolved even though only one is directly treated.

Global. Though the term "global" usually refers to something universal or experienced worldwide, in EFT it refers to problems stated in vague and nonspecific terms, especially in Setup Phrases.

Intensity Meter. The 0-to-10 scale that measures pain, discomfort, anger, frustration, and every other physical or emotional symptom. Intensity can also be indicated with gestures, such as hands held close together (small discomfort) or wide apart (large discomfort).

Mechanical EFT. See Basic Recipe.

Meridians. Invisible channels or pathways through which energy *(chi)* flows in the body. The eight primary meridians pass through five pairs of vital organs, and twelve secondary meridians network to the extremities. The basic premise of EFT is that the cause of every negative emotion and most physical symptoms is a block or disruption in the flow of chi along one or more of the meridians.

Movie Technique, or Watch the Movie Technique. In this process, you review in your mind, as though it were a movie, a bothersome specific event. When intensity comes up, stop and tap on that intensity. When the intensity subsides, continue in your mind with the story. This method has been a mainstay in the toolbox of many EFT practitioners. It may be the most-used EFT technique. For a full description, see the tutorial at www.EFTuniverse.com.

Personal Peace Procedure. An exercise in which you clear problems and release core issues by writing down, as quickly as possible, as many bothersome events from your life that you can remember. Try for at least fifty, or a hundred. Give each event a title, as though it is a book or movie. When the list is complete, begin tapping on the largest issues. Eliminating at least one uncomfortable memory per day (a very conservative schedule) removes at least ninety unhappy events in three months. If you work through two or three per day, it's 180 or 270. For details, see the free Personal Peace Procedure tutorial at www.EFTuniverse.com.

Reminder Phrase. A word, phrase, or sentence that helps the mind focus on the problem being treated. It is used in combination with acupoint tapping.

Setup Phrase, or Setup. An opening statement said at the beginning of each EFT treatment that defines and helps neutralize the problem. In EFT, the standard Setup Phrase is "Even though I have this _____, I fully and completely accept myself."

Story Technique, or Tell the Story Technique. Narrate or tell out loud the story of a specific event dealing with trauma, grief, anger, and so on, and stop to tap whenever the story becomes emotionally intense. Each of the stopping points represents another aspect of the issue that, on occasion, will take you to even deeper issues. This technique is similar to the Movie Technique, except that in the Movie Technique, you simply watch past events unfold in your mind. In the Story Technique, you describe them out loud.

Surrogate or Proxy Tapping. Tapping on yourself on behalf of another person. The person can be present or not. Another way to perform surrogate or proxy tapping is to substitute a photograph, picture, or line drawing for the person and tap on that.

Tail-Enders. The "yes, but" statements that create negative self-talk. When you state a goal or affirmation, tail-enders point the way to core issues.

Tearless Trauma Technique. This is another way of approaching an emotional problem in a gentle way. It involves having the client guess as to the emotional intensity of a past event rather than painfully relive it mentally.

Writings on Your Walls. Limiting beliefs and attitudes that result from cultural conditioning or family attitudes, these are often illogical and harmful yet very strong subconscious influences.

Yin and Yang. See Chi.

EFT Resources

For information about EFT, including a free downloadable Get Started package, go to www.EFTuniverse.com. On this website, you'll find thousands of case histories of people who've used EFT successfully for every conceivable problem. You'll also find practitioner listings, tutorials, books, DVDs, classes, volunteer opportunities, and other resources to allow you to get the most from EFT.

Index

A
acceptance phrase, 45
acupuncture points, 88
Adkins, Maggie, 124
affirmation, 28, 44
anxiety, 10
    progress with, 28
    recovering from, 14
apex effect, 24, 90
aspects, 57
autoimmune disease, 9

B
Basic Recipe, 33
    steps of, 53
Brattberg, Gunilla, 24
breathing and EFT, 28

C
Callahan, Roger, 90
Carter, Stephen, 28
CFIDS, 121

childhood,
    contributing factor to anxiety, 17
chronic fatigue syndrome (CFS), 14, 21, 117
    healing from, 14, 117
    symptoms, 19
    women afflicted by, 21
Collinge, William, 120
core issues, 60

D
depression, 10, 20, 23, 31, 56, 85, 92, 96, 101, 136, 141, 145
    progress with, 28
    recovering from, 25

E
EFT,
    apex effect, 24, 90
    Basic Recipe, 33, 38, 53

Clinical, 33, 38, 76, 86
for pain, 10, 28, 92
Full Basic Recipe, 81, 91
Karate Chop point, 11
9 Gamut Procedure, 84
Reminder Phrase, 52
research, 24, 33
round, 12
Setup Statement, 10, 41
specific events, 55
EFTuniverse.com, 19, 24, 27, 132, 140
emotional upset and stress, 141
energy,
    as constricted, 104
    hygiene, 116
    moving, 96, 122
    obstructed, 42, 97, 99, 101, 116

F
father wound, 150
fear,
    of spiders, 36, 45, 73
    of the future, 147
fibromyalgia,
    accepting, 148
    Chinese medicine, 95, 98, 106, 112, 118
    digestion disturbances, 20, 105, 112
    disharmony of the spirit, 95, 99, 103
    helplessness, 25, 143
    hopelessness, 124, 143
    pain, 9, 10, 20, 22, 92, 96, 133, 140, 145
    progress with, 28
    self-test, 22
    Spleen meridian, 105
    success stories, 28, 133
    three perspectives on, 97
    12-week program, 24, 140, 151
    women afflicted by, 21
forgiveness, adding to Setup, 131
Full Basic Recipe, 41, 79, 81, 88
future, creating positive, 151

G
gamut point, 87
generalization effect, 61

H
Hancock, Salome, 121
Hass, Rue Anne, 95, 118
healing pattern, 120
healing wave, 119
Heart meridian, home of spirit, 109
    insomnia, 105–110
    tapping for issues, 110

I
insomnia, 23, 96, 105, 107, 109
intensity meter, 39

L
Liver meridian, 111
    tapping for issues, 112
low self-esteem, 17, 47, 56, 101, 144, 150
Lukawska, Kristina, 133
Lyme disease, 19, 28, 94, 151

Index

M
Marshall, Sarah L., 14
medications, and NNT and NNH, 26
meridians, 37, 42, 89
    affect the spirit, 103, 105
mother wound, 148

N
9 Gamut Procedure, 84
number needed to harm (NNH), 26
    medications, 26
number needed to treat (NNT), 25
    anxiety, 25
    depression, 25
    medications, 26

P
pain,
    as symptom, 9, 20, 22, 34, 96
    reduction, 10, 26, 33, 136, 140
    tapping for, 10, 28, 92, 104
Personal Peace Procedure, 70, 139
Psychological Reversal, 42, 48
    correcting for, 49

R
Reminder Phrase, 52
round of tapping, 12

S
secondary gain, 48, 146
self-acceptance statement, 10
Selfridge, Nancy, 99
self-test for fibromyalgia, 24
Sequence, the, 50
Setup Statement, 10, 41
    for disharmony of spirit, 103
    sample, 128
side effects,
    and NNT, 27
Small intestine meridian issues, 113
Sore Spot, 80
Spleen meridian, 105
    tapping for issues, 108
stress, 10, 25, 29, 33, 37, 52, 71, 73, 86, 113, 119, 141, 148
Subjective Units of Distress/Discomfort (SUD), 39
SUD scale, 39
symptom severity (SS) scale, 22
symptoms,
    of CSF, 9, 20
    of fibromyalgia, 9, 20

T
tender points, 9
testing results, 38
Top of the Head point, 89
trauma, past, 143

W
'Why Bother' syndrome, 124
Widespread Pain Index (WPI), 22
women, afflicted by fibromyalgia and CFS, 21

A world of wellness at your fingertips!

To see more books in this series of authorized EFT guides, including...

The EFT Manual
EFT for the Highly Sensitive Temperament
EFT for Sports Performance
EFT for Golf
EFT for Love Relationships
EFT for Abundance
EFT for PTSD
EFT for Procrastination
EFT for Back Pain
EFT for Weight Loss

...go to www.EFTuniverse.com